THE PRACTICAL MANAGEMENT OF
EATING & DRINKING DIFFICULTIES
IN CHILDREN

Dedication

This book is dedicated to my parents, Tess and Donald, brothers, Grant and Adam, husband Danny and daughter Bianca, with whom I have shared so many meals.

◆
APRIL WINSTOCK
◆

A registered speech and language therapist, April Winstock has worked in a school for children with moderate learning difficulties, followed by nine years at a district general hospital. She then worked at the Bobath Centre in London and has worked at an RNIB school in Middlesex for several years.

April is currently the speech and language adviser to the Sense Family Centre in London.

She runs courses on the practical management of eating and drinking difficulties in children throughout the UK as well as maintaining her own practice.

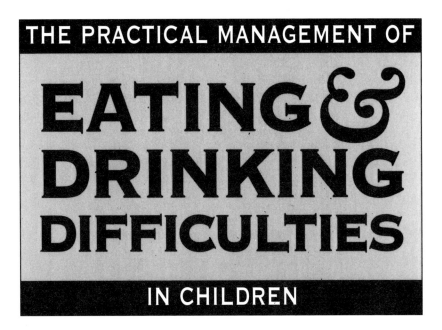

THE PRACTICAL MANAGEMENT OF EATING & DRINKING DIFFICULTIES IN CHILDREN

APRIL WINSTOCK

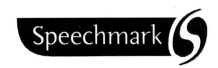

Speechmark Publishing Ltd
Telford Road • Bicester • Oxon OX26 4LQ • UK

For the sake of clarity alone, in this text we have used 'he' to refer to the baby/child and 'she' to refer to the adult.

Published by
Speechmark Publishing Ltd, Telford Road, Bicester, Oxon OX26 4LQ
United Kingdom
www.speechmark.net

002-1718/Printed in the United Kingdom/1030

British Library Cataloguing in Publication Data
Winstock, April
Practical Management of Eating and Drinking Difficulties in Children
1. Title
618.928526

ISBN 0 86388 376 1
(Previously published by Winslow Press Ltd under ISBN 0 86388 123 8)

◆ CONTENTS ◆

LIST OF FIGURES

PREFACE

This book has been written to enable professionals and non-professionals to understand how they can help children who have difficulty in eating and/or drinking. Perhaps we should ask why this is desirable. Children require a balanced and nourishing diet in order to thrive and be healthy. Mealtimes provide an excellent opportunity for practising the patterns of movement of the lips, tongue, jaw, breathing and voice production mechanisms, which influence the development of speech and the control of saliva, as well as enabling the child to improve posture, head control and eye/hand co-ordination. Communication is an integral part of eating and drinking. Mealtimes provide a social setting in which the child is able to express preferences, dislikes and so on. *Everyone* who is involved in preparing and giving meals to children has the potential to help those children to improve their skills in many aspects of their development.

Whilst the text focuses on cerebral palsy the information is also applicable to children who present with a range of disabilities including genetic conditions such as Riley-Day Syndrome, also known as familial dysautonomia, and children who are developmentally delayed.

It is hoped that parents and teachers will have the support of a team of therapists to advise on their children's management. Where this is not available I hope that the information in this book will provide some practical help. However, I would stress the importance of seeking professional help, as a book cannot be a substitute for specialist advice.

The book is designed to be read as a whole. It is important to read the earlier chapters first as they provide the relevant background information that will enable the reader to understand what is suggested later.

I am indebted to all the staff and families at the Bobath Centre, London, which was founded by the late Dr Karel and Mrs Berta Bobath, who helped me to appreciate the importance of asking the questions 'How?', 'Why?' and 'What?' before proceeding with a therapy plan. I hope that those who read this book will do the same.

◆
ACKNOWLEDGEMENTS
◆

I would like to thank the following people, who so kindly read extracts from this book at different stages in its development: Kim Bunker, Jenny Malone, Judith Morris, Freda Smith and Helen Yarrow. In particular, the following people often reread large portions of the book and provided extremely helpful comments: Marian Browne, Lindsay Hardy, Julia Hopkins, Judith Peters, Dr Andy Raffles, Marie Watson, Lindy Wyman and her colleagues from the Sense Family Centre, London. I am extremely grateful to Gerda Fell and Donald Winstock for proofreading so meticulously. I should also like to mention Simmy Fell, who encouraged me through the ups and downs. I am so sorry that he did not live to see the book published.

Thanks are also due to Julie Scott, who so patiently typed (and retyped) the manuscript and to Marie Kennedy, a dietician in Dublin, for the recipe on page 77. Lastly I would like to thank my husband Danny and daughter Bianca for their understanding and patience during the writing of this book.

I hope that all these people realize the importance of their contribution.

CHAPTER ONE

PARENTS & CHILDREN

WHAT comes to mind when you think of eating and drinking? For most of us, eating and drinking evoke pleasant thoughts such as enjoyment and relaxation. Food and drink are certainly sources of pleasure; they satisfy hunger and thirst and provide opportunities for social interaction. We enjoy different tastes, smells and textures of food. We may choose particular crockery and cutlery — coffee does not seem to taste as good when drunk from a paper cup rather than a china cup. We may linger over meals and use them to celebrate important events such as birthdays and anniversaries. As adults, we can often decide what and when we eat. We may skip a meal if we are not hungry, we may eat a sandwich while walking around the shops. Individuals vary a great deal in what they like. Just consider the possibilities when making toast and jam: type and thickness of bread, degree of toasting preferred, brand of margarine/butter, quantity used, flavour of jam selected and amount required. Within the confines of our budget we have a great deal of choice in, for example, what we eat, where we eat, how much we eat and how long we take to eat a meal.

For children who have difficulties in eating and drinking, for their parents and other people who feed them, eating and drinking may not have such positive associations. Mealtimes may be time-consuming and messy. There may be concern about inadequate weight gain. Mealtimes may have involved unpleasant experiences such as vomiting and gagging (retching). The children may even be fearful of eating and drinking. From the children's point of view, meals may be seen as a passive time when they are fed rather than actively eating.

The children may not be able to make choices regarding what they eat or drink, the order in which foods are given, the rate at which they are fed, and so on. We should remember to ask: **'Whose meal is it?'**

First and foremost it is important for everyone involved to consider the needs of the child and his parents. Parents have the responsibility for ensuring adequate nutrition. It is possible to reduce the frequency of changing clothes and bathing without harming the child, but it is **not** acceptable to withhold food and drink.

Parents of a child with eating or drinking difficulties have to deal with an often overwhelming number of visitors, such as therapists, health visitors and social workers, as well as attending numerous hospital appointments. Other family and work commitments may add to demands on their time. Advice should always therefore be discussed with parents to ensure that it is both practical and possible. The following accounts of experiences were written by parents and a grandparent of children with cerebral palsy.

◆ SARAH

Sarah is a six-and-a-half-year-old girl with a severe physical disability. She is unable to do anything physically for herself, she cannot walk, talk, roll or use her arms at all. She makes herself understood with the use of her eyes. She is a happy girl, extremely gregarious, and gets great pleasure from playing with other people.

❝ When Sarah (our first child) was born, we had no idea that she was severely brain damaged. I had had a normal pregnancy and labour and there was no reason to think that anything should be wrong and so we took Sarah home from hospital, naïve and inexperienced in 'parenting' but full of love and joy for her and looking forward to our new life as a family. The first three months were extremely difficult. Sarah hardly ever slept and breast-feeding proved almost impossible, and so, when she was two months old, I started bottle feeding her. It was a very laborious procedure but we persisted, of course, and at least I knew how much she was taking at each feed.

We began to wean her at three months old. I'd seen other babies stick their tongues out when being fed, so I wasn't surprised when Sarah did, although it concerned me that she seemed to push hers out rather more than normal and that more food dribbled out than stayed in, but we carried on assuming that she was just a difficult baby. After a few more weeks, however, it gradually became apparent that something was drastically wrong with Sarah. We began the round of hospital visits and at six and a half months Sarah was diagnosed as having cerebral palsy (spastic quadriplegia). This meant nothing to us except that the word 'spastic' filled us with dread. At that stage feeding problems were the last thing on our minds. Would she walk, talk; would her intellect be impaired? How would we all cope?

Almost immediately we were offered physiotherapy, occupational therapy and hydrotherapy, not a mention of speech and language therapy or help with feeding. As the months went by and the enormity of Sarah's handicap sank in, I kept myself very, very busy. It was, and still is, my way of dealing with the situation. I couldn't have managed without the love and support of my immediate family. My mother, who was also trying to adjust and cope with the emotional stress of her first grandchild being handicapped, looked after Sarah for me to give me a rest. However, one problem kept occurring: no one else could feed her or, more importantly, give her a drink. This meant that the length of time I could leave her was governed by her feeding pattern.

I needed help. Fortunately, at around this time Sarah was accepted at a centre which specializes in treating children with cerebral palsy. They treated Sarah as a whole child and therapy included speech and language as well as physiotherapy and occupational therapy. More importantly, the whole family was involved (including grandparents) with the treatment. The therapists explained what they were doing and why and we were taught how to move, handle and feed Sarah at home. Sarah began drinking from a cup, her chewing and swallowing improved and people other than me were able to feed her, giving me a much-needed rest. None of this happened overnight and now, six years on, we still work on her 'jaw (oral) control' and have periodic intensive sessions on feeding, but the improvements were obvious and without that early intervention I doubt that her feeding would be as good as it is now.

Eating out socially became difficult. Sarah was getting too big to hold and we now had two more children, so at three and a half Sarah obtained a wheelchair. Although emotionally it was quite difficult to come to terms with, it was a breakthrough for us all. People became instantly aware of her problems and, generally speaking, I have found their understanding welcome. She was at the right height at a table, I didn't have to hold her all the time and, most importantly, it gave her dignity.

Problems or situations relating to her feeding arise all the time. Friends or cousins ask why she dribbles. Why do I have to feed her? Some spend the whole of the meal reminding me that a piece of food has fallen out! No one at Sunday School or Rainbow Brownies is confident enough to feed her and so outings are out of the question, unless I go along as well.

As mentioned before, Sarah is a happy child. Even this occasionally causes problems. She gets great pleasure from eating with friends or at parties. However, she smiles so much it is almost impossible for her to eat. Looking back over the last six or seven years I remember with joy and pride the achievements: our first meal in a restaurant with her, her first day at school, not having to prepare food in advance and especially for her, ordering a 'take-away' knowing she would be able to eat it. If anyone offers to feed her while I am around I accept now, but I have to leave the room, because in my eyes no one can feed her as well as me! **"**
Helen

◆ A GRANDMA'S PERSPECTIVE

❝ **I have** written a few paragraphs on how a grandma can help when there is a child with special needs in the family. Since feeding is often a problem it is a good idea to set aside a day to prepare complete little meals for freezing so that, when there is a particularly busy day, Mum or Dad can just grab one from the freezer.

Also, to help with washing and keeping clothes clean, making bibs in jolly, patterned material backed with dark-coloured towelling to ensure that liquids don't penetrate to the chest is helpful. If you sew a small piece of Velcro to secure it round the neck then you don't have to drag the bib over the head. (See Figure 1.) As you can see, there is a deep pocket at the bottom to catch food. On special occasions like birthdays and Christmas I like to make special ones in appropriate material, adding bows and motifs etc.

There were only three pieces of kitchen equipment which I found essential — a simple blender, a microwave and a mincer. I didn't use foil at all (with the microwave in mind) but plastic freezer bags, labelled in different colours, denoting savoury or sweet meals and freezer separating paper. This was used to wrap the food in at the outset, as it was all right to place it on the

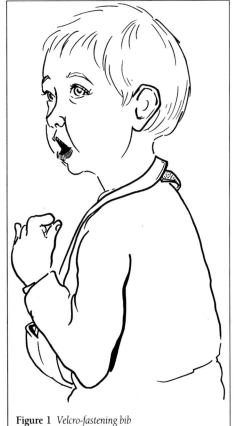

Figure 1 *Velcro-fastening bib*

child's dish in the microwave. I used a large *Tupperware*-type box to contain the individually wrapped bags.

Right at the beginning of the cooking session I would make a mound of instant mash potato (invaluable and has all the right vitamins!), at the very least a pint of white sauce (any over can be frozen for next time) and a pile of grated cheese.

I don't feel there is a need to be too adventurous and my meals were often made from: corned beef, chicken (very versatile), fish— ask the fishmonger for the tail end as there are far less bones (incidentally, in some supermarkets they actually sell minced fish), all sorts of vegetables, finely minced beef steak, as well as puréed prunes, apricots, stewed peeled apples, custard and chocolate sauce. Incidentally, onions, mustard and tomato purée used with a light hand make meals more interesting — savoury that is!

It is also important to buy good-quality bread, as this tends not to cling to the roof of the mouth. Some children find bread difficult to shift and can get quite distressed. It is impossible to give specific amounts for menus or recipes as children's appetites vary and I often adapted recipes and then divided what I had cooked into Sarah-sized meals. ❞
Freda

◆ LIANNE

❝ **Lianne** was born two months premature after a very difficult pregnancy: I spent the last three months on bed rest in the antenatal ward. Lianne weighed just under four pounds and looked perfectly well and normal. She passed all tests performed on her and did not need ventilating or any other help from the Special Care Unit. I was able to breast-feed her from day one and she thrived on it, and gained weight dramatically. After we were both discharged from the post-natal ward on the tenth day I presumed I would settle down to a normal, uncomplicated life. Little did I know what lay in store.

I did not expect life to be easy. After all, I was having to feed Lianne every three hours, day and night, which in itself was exhausting. I also had Natalie at home, my other daughter, who was 18 months old when I went into hospital and was now 21 months and not very happy with her mother who had decided (in her mind) to live elsewhere for a long time.

Until Lianne was two months old things went relatively smoothly, but then she began screaming day and night. Nothing would console her. To begin with I naturally thought it was something quite minor like colic — but it continued day after day until I became a physical and emotional wreck. She was being routinely checked every six weeks as she was premature and I was continually reassured that she was developing normally. After months of being told the same thing and me noticing lots of changes I didn't think were normal, I asked for a second opinion and at nine months of age Lianne was diagnosed as having cerebral palsy.

Throughout those months I continued breast-feeding her, not out of choice but because she refused any type of bottle or feeding cup and any other type of milk. Amazingly, at nine months of age she weighed 18 pounds. Today Lianne is approaching five years and weighs little over 20 pounds! Looking back I am amazed I ever got through those early months. If only the professionals had listened to my concerns. Obviously, it would not have helped Lianne's condition, but it would certainly have helped me.

By the time she was diagnosed I had managed to get her established on puréed baby foods but had found the whole process very distressing, as she was so difficult to feed. Now I knew why. Whilst she sucked the breast easily, she was unable to suck a teat or take food from a spoon. Consequently, feeding was a long, laborious job, not at all the pleasurable time I had had with Natalie. I thought help would be at hand once Lianne's diagnosis had been made. Sadly, this was not the case. Physiotherapy did not start until she was over one year of age and speech and language therapy, including help with feeding, not until much later.

Today, Lianne has severe cerebral palsy affecting all four limbs. Consequently, she is unable to sit, crawl, walk or talk, being totally dependent on others. She is, however, mentally bright and has a wicked sense of humour! Despite her low weight she does have an amazing appetite, eating three good meals a day, plus biscuits and treats in between. She will attempt to eat almost anything, but for safety reasons her meals are generally mashed or semi-puréed. Any lumps cause her to gag or choke, which is distressing to both of us.

It takes a long time to feed Lianne, especially at teatime, when new foods are tried. Lianne is now at school, so a good half-hour is set aside to give her breakfast and anything between one and two hours for tea. She enjoys her meals immensely but I still find the whole process takes a good portion of my time out of the day. She attempts to eat mashed food and manages very well, but this takes even longer. She usually returns home from school very tired, so this is done only at weekends. She likes to have the same food as her older sister and always enjoys it when this happens. You do need plenty of time and patience.

Lianne is fed either in her specialized chair or, when tired, on my lap, which she always finds easier — and so do I! Her athetoid movements are worse in her arms so splints are applied so that she can hold onto a grab bar on her table-top, which generally helps her to balance and makes feeding Lianne a lot easier. Her chewing action has improved slowly over the years, but she will also suck food off the spoon and foods she finds difficult to chew are swallowed whole! For instance, she adores satsumas, but can find the segments difficult to chew and sometimes they disappear down the back of her throat, causing me a good amount of alarm, which she finds hilarious! Caution is needed!

Lianne now drinks from a *Doidy* cup, which is one of our most valued pieces of equipment. After finally packing in breast-feeding (when Lianne had reached one!) and after numerous attempts with different bottles and beakers, she would only ever drink properly from a *Maws* spouted beaker (they have since changed the design) and the *Doidy* cup. She enjoys most juices, even water, just as long as it isn't milk!

She loves going out for meals, which isn't a common occurrence, but when we go into *McDonalds* or somewhere similar she shrieks with delight. She loves chips, and finds them quite manageable, but the burgers are quite difficult for her. She tries very hard, even though the food is normally stone cold, but loves the whole experience. I still find it quite difficult taking her into public places. Public reaction can be upsetting but sometimes understandable, when they see a child gagging on a piece of hamburger!

Natalie is now six years old and understands a lot about her sister's condition. She obviously finishes her meals a lot sooner than Lianne and will then want something else, like yogurt or fruit, but has learnt to sit out of Lianne's sight with them, as Lianne will then want what she has and refuse to eat any more of her dinner! I often think how lovely it would be for us just to sit round the table and all eat at the same time, but this is very rare.

Feeding Lianne is not always easy and it is very time-consuming, but I think I am at least fortunate in that she has a very good appetite and, despite her low weight gain, enjoys her food and has always eaten well.

Handy hints

1 Seek advice from professionals and especially from parents with children who have special needs. Their advice, I have found, is invaluable.
2 I find it easier to have plenty of frozen meals at hand. Sometimes, if we have a rare take-away, which Lianne is unable to manage, a ready-prepared meal will be there.
3 Invest in a good food processor or food mixer, so meals can be made in bulk and frozen.
4 Have plenty of bibs or children's painting aprons. The waterproof ones are best so that clothes underneath are not ruined. Keep lots of kitchen paper at hand to tuck around the neck, or to mop up spills.
5 Try and make feeding a relaxed, happy occasion, which I know is not always easy to do and is sometimes impossible, but if the child senses you are concerned and worried it will only make feeding more difficult.

6 Have everything ready so when you sit down you do not have to keep popping back to the kitchen to get something. This only unsettles the child.
7 I have found with Lianne that she will eat far better in a quiet atmosphere than if there is a lot of noise going on around her.

Incidentally, at school Lianne is in the nursery class, consisting of five pupils, and they have their lunch in class. The staff feel that the school hall would be too noisy and unsettling for them. **99**

Kim

It is essential that people involved in feeding children *listen* to parents, grandparents and other adults who are familiar with those children. Their knowledge, feelings and concerns play an important part in planning therapy for their children.

◆

CHAPTER TWO

HOW EATING & DRINKING NORMALLY DEVELOP

◆

BEFORE considering the eating and drinking difficulties experienced by children with special needs, it is important to understand how the infant normally acquires the necessary skills. Please note that children's development varies a great deal and *all age levels used below are approximate.* From before birth the baby experiences sucking and swallowing of amniotic fluid (the liquid that surrounds the baby in the womb).

SUCKING

From birth the infant's *rooting reflex* enables him to locate the nipple or teat. Once the baby latches on, he starts to suck and swallow easily and rhythmically. From birth the baby automatically co-ordinates sucking and swallowing with his breathing. Breathing normally stops momentarily during a swallow. The strength and speed of the sucking will be determined by the baby's degree of hunger, wakefulness, milk supply and so on. The baby is usually fed in a semi-reclining position. At this stage the anatomical structures of the mouth and neck make this both safe and comfortable. The baby's early sucking consists of a forward – backward tongue movement and simultaneous up – down jaw movement. In the first few months of life the suck is immediately followed by a swallow and this 'unit' is known as a 'suckle'. Lip closure is not always complete and some liquid loss may occur, for example if the milk flows very quickly. Dribbling is common.

A young baby will gag (retch) easily. The gag reflex is a normal protective mechanism present throughout life. It is particularly sensitive in the first few months after birth. It becomes less sensitive when the baby starts to chew (between seven and nine months). The most important protective mechanism is the *cough reflex*, which is also present throughout life. It involves closure of the vocal cords within the larynx (voice box) to prevent food/liquid entering the airway.

WEANING

In the west it is customary to wean babies on to semi-solids from three–four months. This occurs much later in many other countries. The baby will usually be sat more upright for feeding at this stage. First weaning foods are typically baby rice, liquidized fruit and vegetables. The baby's initial reaction appears to be one of spitting out the food as he uses his habitual forward – backward tongue movement. The baby sucks food from the spoon (usually plastic and deep bowled) helped by the feeder, who tends to tip the spoon into the child's mouth. This is important because at this stage the baby is not easily able to use his lips well enough to remove food placed horizontally in the mouth. With practice the baby's tongue-tip *gradually* starts to move upwards in the mouth and his jaw moves less. This period is important, but it tends to be messy as the baby develops preferences and the spitting out becomes deliberate and enjoyable!

From about four months the baby starts mouthing; that is, putting his hands, toys, clothes and feet into his mouth. This exploration teaches the baby about different objects, tastes and textures. He also discovers his body and learns, for example, that 'Those toes belong to me!'

Chewing

Mouthing provides useful pre-chewing experience. By six months the baby can sit quite well and has good control of his head and trunk (body). This is necessary for the development of the more complex mouth movements involved in chewing and babbling.

The baby will usually be seated in a high chair with perhaps padding and a tray to provide support. However, in some cultures it is customary to sit on the floor to eat, so that babies are more likely to be fed on a lap or propped up on cushions. Anatomical changes between the ages of four and six months mean that swallowing safely requires fine co-ordination. Upright seating from this age is important for safety and comfort!

◆ PRACTICAL EXERCISE 1

This is to help you discover the importance of how you are positioned when eating/drinking. You need a biscuit and a glass of water.

1 Sit upright. Eat some biscuit and then drink some water.
2 Repeat this leaning backwards while keeping your head upright.
3 Repeat this while tipping your head back.

Note how much more difficult it is to eat and drink when your body, and *particularly when your head, is tipped back.*

From about six months, teeth start to come through. Dribbling is common during teething, although it decreases as the baby's physical development matures. More solid food such as mashed banana is introduced, although the baby may have initial difficulty with lumps.

◆ PRACTICAL EXERCISE 2

This is to enable you to experience how your mouth reacts to different textures. You need two spoonfuls of *smooth* custard, yogurt (*without* fruit pieces) or similar and one raisin or sultana.

1 Eat one spoonful of the custard or yogurt and think about how you do it. In particular note how you use your lips and tongue.
2 Place the raisin or sultana in the second spoonful of custard or yogurt and then eat it.

Which was easier? Most people find eating just the custard or yogurt on its own easier. In order to manage the second spoonful you need to use your tongue to feel for the fruit, move it and then store it in the side of your mouth while you swallowed the custard or yogurt. You *then* chew the raisin. This is a complex process involving sensation (feeling), perception (interpreting feeling) and co-ordinated tongue and lip movements — no wonder many six-month-olds find manufactured 'Junior' foods containing a combination of textures difficult to eat.

Munching

The first stage in chewing begins at about six months. If a rusk is placed *to the side* of the baby's mouth, the baby will start to bite up and down (munch) on it. Once softened, the rusk moves onto the tongue and sucking commences. Eating firmer foods provides practice in biting off pieces of food. However, it can be dangerous to give babies hard foods, such as raw carrot and apple, which do not dissolve once bitten and may cause choking. For this reason babies should *not* be given such hard foods, or be left alone with food.

Between seven and nine months the tongue begins to move sideways, but it is only from about 12 months that the child can transfer food from the centre of the tongue to either side of the mouth. Transferring food from side to side without pausing in the centre develops gradually. The lips also become more skilful as the baby develops. The upper lip *actively* removes food from the spoon from about nine months, so that the feeder does not need to tip the spoon. By this stage food is usually thicker and the spoon is flatter, thereby making this action easier. By 18 months the baby can chew with his lips closed, although intermittent mouth opening is common except during swallowing, when the lips close, forming a seal. Between 12 and 18 months rotatory jaw and tongue movements are seen. By two years the child can use fairly precise tongue movements for chewing. Food and saliva may still be lost until about two years of age owing to incomplete lip closure.

◆ PRACTICAL EXERCISE 3

This is to increase your awareness of lip closure during eating. You need a slice of bread and a mirror.

While looking in the mirror, bite off a piece of bread and watch yourself chew.

Notice how you *do not* maintain lip closure throughout (unless you are really concentrating on doing so). Watch people eating and notice how often they close their mouth. Adults usually teach children to chew discreetly.

DRINKING

Bottle/breast (see 'Sucking' above)

Many British children are given a cup by the age of 12 months, although a night-time or early morning bottle or breast-feed may still be offered. In other countries bottles or the breast are routinely offered to children for much longer.

Cup

A cup may be introduced from four to six months. A training cup is often offered at first to reduce spillage. It is held for the baby who initially uses a forward – backward tongue movement with up – down jaw movement, resulting in some liquid loss. At about 12 months the tongue may protrude slightly beneath the cup to provide some stability. At 18 months the child may bite on the edge of the cup to stabilize it. He can drink in long sequences and can hold liquid in the mouth once the cup is removed. His top lip closes on the edge of the cup and the tongue neither protrudes from the mouth nor rests beneath the cup. From two years, a more mature up – down sucking pattern is used and the child can now keep his jaw still without biting the cup.

Straw

With the invention and popularity of the juice carton, babies as young as 12 months have learnt to use a straw. However, it is important to remember that they are already able to use a cup quite well by this stage, so that the straw is not used instead of a cup.

FURTHER CONSIDERATIONS

Behaviour

From the age of two to three years food refusal and fussiness is quite common. Advice is available through health visitors or general practitioners.

Cultural/religious aspects

There are many variations in the way people of different religious/cultural groups eat and drink. Certain foods may be prohibited. Weaning may occur much later. The way in which people are seated may vary. Utensils may be different or may not be used. In some cultures only the right hand may be used for eating. This has implications for the child with a physical disability who may have to use his left ('unclean') hand for eating. It is important to be aware of people's attitudes when discussing possible changes.

◆ SAFETY — IMPORTANT INFORMATION

Throughout these early years all babies and children should be closely supervised when eating or drinking.

◆ SUMMARY

By two–three years the child can chew and drink using efficient tongue, lip and jaw movements. His co-ordination of eating, drinking and breathing is well established. When the synchronization is disturbed, as when, for example, the child drinks too quickly, an effective cough normally clears the airway. The child can use his hands, a spoon and fork and is largely independent, although help and supervision are essential. A common feature of eating behaviour in this age group is fussiness and some degree of food (seldom drink) refusal. Toddlers tend to prefer frequent snacks to three meals a day. They are often very active and may not readily sit down at mealtimes. They will often wish to eat only a few foods, which usually include biscuits, chocolate and crisps of some sort! Understandably, parental concern may result in two-year-olds dictating what and when they want to eat or drink. This can get out of control and professional help is sometimes required to help parents deal with such behaviour. In most cases these problems are successfully resolved. However, where problems are causing concern, parents should seek advice from their health visitor or general practitioner.

		KEY STAGES IN THE DEVELOPMENT OF EATING AND DRINKING SKILLS					
	Position of baby	**Food/Fluid**	**Eating pattern**	**Drinking pattern**	**Self-feeding**	**Communication**	**Food–related play**
Birth to 3 months	Semi-reclining.	Milk, water, well-diluted baby juices.		Sucking. Forward – backward tongue movement with simultaneous up – down jaw movement. Easy, rhythmical movement. Gag reflex very sensitive.		Cries, gurgles, eye and facial expression, body movements.	
3 to 6 months	More upright — requires support.	Milk, water, well-diluted baby juices. Smooth, liquidized semi-solids introduced.	Initially 'spits out' food, using habitual forward – backward tongue movement. Dribbles. Gradually learns to suck food from a spoon.	Cup introduced.		Uses eyes and voice. Takes turns in vocalization. Body movement, facial expression.	Mouths, hands, toys, clothes, feet and so on.
6 to 9 months	Upright — may or may not require support.	Can now take mashed foods. Finger foods such as rusks are introduced *under supervision*.	More vertical tongue-tip and less jaw movement. Able to bite food placed to *sides* of mouth. Sucks once food gets onto tongue.	Initial liquid loss common as jaw moves up and down and tongue moves forward and backward. Tongue may protrude slightly.	Can hold bottle without help. Puts hands to cup. Picks up pieces of food.	Vocalizes to attract attention. Babbles.	Enjoys babbling with a mouthful of food. Enjoys feeling food.
9 to 12 months	Sits upright independently, therefore *able to develop independent use of arms and hands*.	Firmer food is chopped and more varieties can be held in the hand. Food given by spoon is thicker. A flatter bowled spoon is often used.	Tongue able to transfer food from side to side within mouth. Gag reflex becomes less sensitive though *still present and necessary*. Upper lip active in removing food from spoon.	Tongue moves forward and backward. It may protrude beneath the cup to provide stability.	Allows adult to supervise and control feeding. Able to finger-feed. Plays with food. Can hold a spoon, but with poor control. Puts hands to cup. May try to hold it.	Shakes head for 'no'. Points. Imitates sounds. Uses jargon (sentence-like sounds).	Enjoys playing with food: prodding, spreading, squeezing it and so on.
12 to 18 months		Offered an increasing variety of firmer foods.	Able to chew efficiently with lateral and rotatory tongue/jaw movement. Lip closure is intermittent whilst chewing, but occurs when swallowing.	At 18 months the child may bite on edge of cup to stabilize jaw. Upper lip closes on edge of cup, providing better seal. Tongue does not protrude and less jaw movement is seen.	Child able to bring filled spoon to mouth, but turns it over en route. Finger-feeds well. Holds cup but often spills drink.	Child using some meaningful words. Imitates noises and words. Points and gestures.	Pretends to feed himself/another person/large doll, teddy.

The Practical Management of Eating & Drinking Difficulties in Children

	Position of child	Food/Fluid	Eating pattern	Drinking pattern	Self-feeding	Communication	Food–related play
18 to 24 months		Able to chew firmer foods.	Able to use a controlled, sustained bite on a biscuit. Can chew with lips closed. May lose food or saliva while chewing.	Uses an up – down sucking pattern with the cup between the lips. Internal jaw stabilization developing, so no longer needs to bite edge of cup.	Gradually gets spoon to mouth without turning it. Becomes independent with spoon. Moderate spillage. Lifts cup to mouth and may tip it too much, causing spillage. Gradually progresses to releasing cup without spillage.	Child's vocabulary increases. Begins to imitate and spontaneously use two-word combinations.	Pretends to feed toys such as small-scale dolls.
24 to 36 months			Eats well, with little spillage. Some assistance needed.	Drinks well, with little spillage.	Uses fork.	Child uses short sentences to express likes, dislikes and so on. Often very strong-willed and prone to tantrums.	Enjoys playing with tea-set, pots and pans.
36 to 48 months					Spreads butter on bread with knife.		Enjoys more elaborate 'pretend' play such as going shopping, cooking, feeding himself and toys. Enjoys helping adults to mix and stir food.
48 to 60 months					Cuts with knife.		Elaborate 'pretend' play continues with increasing complexity.

CHAPTER THREE

COMMUNICATION AT MEALTIMES

IMAGINE that you are six months old. You are hungry but do not like what you have been given. What do you do? Cry? Spit it out? Try to get out of your chair? Eat a bit, then moan? Look at the dessert that is on a nearby table? I am sure that you can think of more possibilities, and if you were older, say twelve months, you would have even more ways of expressing your disgust, such as shaking your head, pointing to the cupboard because you remember where the biscuits are kept, pushing the bowl onto the floor or throwing food to the dog! It is very important to understand how babies and young children normally communicate at mealtimes. There is often a physical closeness, especially when the child is young. The child becomes familiar with the carer's face, body, voice and particular smell. This enables a trusting relationship to develop and is a focal part of bonding, the emotional closeness that exists between an adult and a baby.

For older children and adults, mealtimes provide an ideal opportunity to share news, discuss everyday matters and appreciate other people's viewpoints. Children learn how to take turns and to share. New vocabulary is acquired along with table manners! When children have difficulty in eating and drinking, they should still be part of family mealtimes. They can benefit from the social aspects of eating together, even if their physical disabilities prevent them from eating the same food as their family or friends. *Good communication makes mealtimes easier and easier mealtimes promote improved communication.* Children are more likely to make progress in a relaxed atmosphere and improved communication should reduce misunderstanding and frustration for everyone. It is important to try to see mealtimes as being as pleasurable as possible.

In order to communicate as effectively as possible the child should be well positioned, that is with an upright head and body. See Chapter 5 on positioning for further information. It is important to be aware that people should position themselves (as well as any pictures or symbols that are used) in such a way as to reduce the likelihood of the child changing *his* position in order to see *them*. For example, some children may go into a pattern of extension (pushing back) if they have to look *up* to see something or someone. Television as a routine mealtime companion can be extremely distracting and is not recommended.

We need to consider how non-speaking children may express their feelings towards the food or drink offered. They are able to do so using a variety of non-verbal behaviour. Let us look more closely at what this includes. There are four main ways in which non-verbal behaviour can be expressed: (1) using eyes; (2) using voice; (3) using mouth and facial movements; and (4) using gestures or body movements. There is *clearly overlap between these*, and many movements occur simultaneously. However, for clarity I have divided them up somewhat artificially. Infants and babies often communicate to express needs, likes or dislikes. *Feeding a child provides an ideal opportunity for communication between the child and his feeder.*

A child will often use combinations of movement, eye gaze and vocalization to express his needs, such as gurgling while reaching for food that he is looking at.

Being familiar with and learning to observe non-verbal behaviour is important in developing the communication skills of the non-speaking child. Whereas children normally have a large repertoire of well co-ordinated movements, the child with cerebral palsy has much less well controlled movement patterns. What is more, these movements are often involuntary, inconsistent, poorly graded and lack refinement, so that they are easy to misinterpret. The child often has great difficulty in making eye contact with the feeder, let alone the food and drink.

Mealtimes are very stimulating occasions — consider the smells, sight of food, and sounds of preparation and the feelings of hunger and anticipation. This excitement often makes the child with cerebral palsy stiffer and he may push backwards in an abnormal pattern of movement unintentionally. It is easy to assume that this movement is being used to refuse food when in fact it might mean quite the opposite. How can we improve our own observation skills in order to help non-verbal children learn to communicate more effectively? The following chart is designed to help you achieve this. Do not try to fill it in at one mealtime. It is difficult to observe so many behaviours at once, especially when you are also trying to feed the child. It might be helpful to video a mealtime, then analyse it later. Filling in the chart with another person is also useful. It is quite likely that there will be disagreement regarding your observations and their interpretation. Do not worry about these discrepancies, rather look upon them as points for further observation and discussion.

This photocopiable chart is designed to help you become more familiar with how the child lets you know what he likes to eat/drink and how he likes to be fed or helped during mealtimes.

Do not try to fill it all in at one mealtime. Look at specific parts over several meals. You might like to video a mealtime and look at it later. You may find it helpful to share your observations with someone else. Where your views differ, use those as points for discussion and further observation.

Finding out about how the child communicates will help not only mealtime enjoyment but many other activities as well, such as playing and dressing.

Child's name

Age

Feeder's name

Location (Home, school etc)

Dates/time period of observation

The child may well have his own ways of communicating,
which you should add in the spaces provided below.

	To express a preference/like/'more'	**To express rejection/dislike/'no more'**
Use of eyes	◆ Look at or for feeder, food or utensil ◆ Look from feeder to food or drink ◆ Look at place associated with food ◆ Look or point with eyes towards a preferred food, container, picture of food and so on. ◆ Express emotion, such as wide-eyed delight ◆ _____ ◆ _____	◆ Look away from feeder, food or utensil ◆ Close eyes ◆ Blink ◆ Look from feeder to preferred food/drink or other source of activity such as a toy ◆ Express emotion; for example, screw up eyes with distaste ◆ _____ ◆ _____
Use of voice	◆ Contented coo/gurgle ◆ Laugh/giggle/squeal ◆ Specific sound meaning 'yes' ◆ Excited, breathy voice ◆ Intonation conveying desire ◆ _____ ◆ _____	◆ Cry — general or a special cry ◆ Fuss, whine, grunt ◆ Specific sound meaning 'no' ◆ Intonation conveying displeasure ◆ _____ ◆ _____ ◆ _____
Use of mouth/facial movements	◆ Open mouth ◆ Feeding movements such as sucking ◆ Increased dribbling ◆ Stronger, faster sucking ◆ Smile ◆ Happy expression ◆ Blow raspberries, smack lips ◆ _____ ◆ _____ ◆ _____	◆ Close mouth or refuse to open it ◆ Do not swallow — may hold food in mouth, let food fall out ◆ Use slow, weak suck ◆ Frown ◆ Sad expression, pout ◆ Gag, cough, choke ◆ Spit out food ◆ Bite on spoon ◆ _____

The child may well have his own ways of communicating, which
you should add in the spaces provided below.

	To express a preference/like/'more'	*To express rejection/dislike/'no more'*
Use of gestures/ body movements	◆ Move towards food/drink/feeder ◆ Reach for food/drink/feeder ◆ Point to food/drink/feeder/symbols ◆ Move hands to mouth, suck hands ◆ Nod head for 'yes' ◆ Wave arms and kick legs ◆ Wriggle body ◆ Stiffen ◆ Play with food ◆ _____ ◆ _____ ◆ _____ ◆ _____ ◆ _____ ◆ _____ ◆ _____	◆ Push back with head and/or hips ◆ Stiffen ◆ Slide down in chair ◆ Get out of chair ◆ Pull away from spoon or food ◆ Push food, spoon, bowl away/off table ◆ Hide face ◆ Point to *preferred* food or source of activity, such as a toy ◆ Shake head for 'no' ◆ Wave arms and kick legs ◆ Wriggle body ◆ Play with food ◆ Point to symbols, pictures ◆ _____ ◆ _____ ◆ _____

TYPE OF COMMUNICATION	USE OF EYES	USE OF VOICE/ SPEECH	USE OF MOUTH/ FACIAL MOVEMENTS	USE OF GESTURES/ BODY MOVEMENTS	OTHER, SUCH AS BREATHING RATE
◆ *I want to eat* (When food is present or at a regular mealtime)					
◆ *I want to eat* (When food is not present)					
◆ *I like/want a particular food*					
◆ *I do not like/want a particular food*					

The Practical Management of Eating & Drinking Difficulties in Children

TYPE OF COMMUNICATION	USE OF EYES	USE OF VOICE/ SPEECH	USE OF MOUTH/ FACIAL MOVEMENTS	USE OF GESTURES/ BODY MOVEMENTS	OTHER, SUCH AS BREATHING RATE
◆ **I need a slower pace for eating/ drinking** (or a brief pause)					
◆ **I want you to speed up the pace for eating/ drinking**					
◆ **I am ready for the next spoonful**					
◆ **I would like to choose which food** (or liquid) **I want next**					

The Practical Management of Eating & Drinking Difficulties in Children

TYPE OF COMMUNICATION	USE OF EYES	USE OF VOICE/ SPEECH	USE OF MOUTH/ FACIAL MOVEMENTS	USE OF GESTURES/ BODY MOVEMENTS	OTHER, SUCH AS BREATHING RATE
◆ *I am still hungry* (or thirsty) ***and want to continue eating/drinking***					
◆ *I no longer wish to eat or drink*					
◆ *I like a particular temperature of food/drink*					
◆ *I dislike a particular temperature of food/drink*					

19

The Practical Management of Eating & Drinking Difficulties in Children

◆ SOCIAL ASPECTS	◆ NOTES
Where else does _____ eat?	
When _____ eats elsewhere, are the same conditions present?	
If not, how and why do they differ? And what effect does this have on _____ ?	
Who usually feeds _____ ? Is anyone else present?	
How do you/other people usually respond to _____'s 'messages'?	

◆ POSITION	◆ NOTES
How is _____ positioned at mealtimes?	
What support is given? What position is the head in?	
Where do you sit — and why?	
Can _____ see your face at mealtimes?	

◆ SENSORY	◆ NOTES
What distractions are there at mealtimes?	
(a) Sounds, such as food preparation, other children, radio	
(b) Sights, such as other people, television	
How does _____ react to these stimuli?	

◆ *Summarize your observations*

◆ *What changes could be made to make communication easier?*

◆ *If the child was going to be fed by someone unfamiliar, what advice would you give her and why?*

Having filled in the chart, you should have a fairly good idea of the ways in which the child is able to tell you how he feels about mealtimes. You can now try to create situations in which he is able to indicate preferences and so on. For example, if you show him two foods or a spoon and a cup, he could perhaps use his eyes to scan the objects and then look longer at his preferred choice, a particular food or drink. It is important to offer choices in such a way that the child is able to respond — ask his therapists or teachers or parents for advice. It is particularly important that items are presented or held at the appropriate angle, distance from the child, height and so on, or he may be unable to communicate effectively. Problems can arise, as in the case, for example, of objects being held up too high so that the child lifts his head, leading to him pushing back his entire body.

Do ensure that you *only offer a choice if you are prepared to act on what the child 'tells' you.* I remember hearing of a child being offered two different drinks; his feeder asked, "Which do you want — orange or blackcurrant?" The child looked deliberately at the blackcurrant drink. The feeder said, "Blackcurrant? You had that yesterday — have orange today." Imagine being asked if you wanted milk in your coffee, replying "Yes", then being told, "You had milk in it this morning — so have it without milk now!" This child was unable to speak and his only means of communication was 'eye pointing'; that is, by looking at what he wanted. He would not have been able to insist on *his* choice as *we* would insist on the milk in our coffee.

The ways in which the child communicates at mealtimes can and should be utilized in as many other situations as possible, as with eye pointing to one of two items of clothing, waiting for the child to make a sound to indicate that you should turn over a page in a book, looking at one of two people to choose who is going to bath him, and so on.

Try *not to anticipate the child's every need.* Give him *time*, watch him carefully and *wait for him to initiate* the conversation. Your speech and language therapist will be able to advise you further.

◆ **REMEMBER**

Good communication makes mealtimes easier and easier mealtimes promote improved communication.

CHAPTER FOUR

THE LINK BETWEEN PHYSICAL DEVELOPMENT AND EATING & DRINKING SKILLS

OUR muscles work in groups which respond to the brain by working together in patterns rather than as single muscle units. Even when we are at rest they are active or in a state of partial contraction which is known as 'muscle tone'. Many factors may affect or alter muscle tone. These may be *physical*, as when changing position or being moved quickly, *environmental* — for example, noisy surroundings or the movement of people in and out of a room — or *emotional*, such as fear or excitation. We are not normally aware of how our muscle tone is regulated. Under normal circumstances it is high enough to maintain our posture against gravity (or we would be unable to get up from the ground) but not so high as to interfere with movement. By studying how movement normally develops, we see how the development of head control is the basis for all our activities and movements. The head contains sense organs for vision, hearing, taste, smell and balance. Whenever we move, we adjust the position of the head, holding it steady in mid-line to the body, that is not tilted forwards, backwards or sideways.

Cerebral palsy is a disorder of posture and movement resulting from damage to the brain either before, during or shortly after birth. It is a non-progressive but changing condition. The child with cerebral palsy usually has poor head control related to abnormal patterns of movement governed by disordered messages from the brain. For example, some children with cerebral palsy frequently push back into a pattern of extension; that is, straightening and possibly scissoring (crossing) the legs, arching the back and tipping back the head. This clearly has an adverse effect on many skills, including how the child breathes, eats and drinks. The child with cerebral palsy has abnormal muscle tone which makes normal co-ordinated movement difficult.

Increased muscle tone (spasticity) is felt as resistance to being moved. To the adult, the child may appear stiff. Movements are difficult and the child may tend to stay in a particular posture, such as stiffly extended (straight) or flexed (bent). (See Figures 2 and 3.) The child with spasticity may not be able to open his mouth very easily and is often sensitive to touch around the mouth. His lips and cheeks may feel tight and move in a limited way. The child's tongue may appear stiff and bunched up towards the roof of the mouth and its movement limited, or the tongue may move too much and be seen pushing forwards excessively.

Reduced or low muscle tone (hypotonicity) describes a state where the muscle tone is too low and the child feels floppy. The child has no stable point from which to start a movement. He may feel like jelly and heavy in your arms. He has difficulty in maintaining a position unaided; for example, when sitting he may collapse to one side. His head often flops forward or backward and his mouth may open, with tongue protruding. His tongue may look too large because it is floppy.

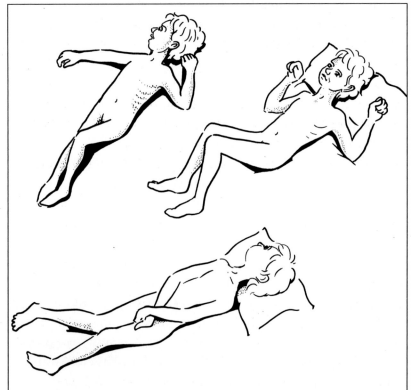

Figure 2 *The mainly extended child*
Note: the head is tipped back; the legs turn in and may cross; the back is arched; the mouth is often open; the arms may be stretched out or bent up.

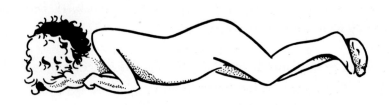

Figure 3 *The mainly flexed child*
Note: the head is forward and facing down; the back is rounded; the arms are pulled up to the chin; the legs are bent and may be pulled up towards the stomach.

◆ **PRACTICAL EXERCISE 4**

This exercise helps you see how your tongue's appearance can change.

Look in a mirror and put out your tongue. See how stiff/floppy you can make it and observe how its appearance changes. Note how it appears to be larger when it is floppy.

Fluctuating tone describes tone which changes rapidly.

Athetoid describes a child with no fixed posture. As in hypotonia, the child with athetosis lacks a stable base from which to start movement. Eating and drinking difficulties are often seen in the child with athetosis because he has poor head control. Involuntary movements are seen which are uncontrolled and excessive. The child may find it nearly impossible to be still. There are often involuntary movements of the face, known as grimacing. The child may wish to smile or talk but the attempt results in excessive, uncontrolled facial movements. The effort involved in attempting movement and speaking often leads to further disorganization of movement. However, if the trunk is stabilized, his movement will improve. He will nevertheless still have difficulty in achieving controlled, graded movements. This may lead to problems such as overtilting a cup, overreaching for a spoon and poor control of jaw, tongue and lips for eating and drinking. The child's head is often tipped back (extended), the mouth opens wide and the tongue protrudes excessively — this is a tongue thrust, which will be discussed later (see page 61).

Ataxic describes a child who lacks balance and who is jerky and unsteady. His movements are poorly timed, graded (incorrectly judged) and directed.

Without treatment, the child with cerebral palsy has no alternative to abnormal patterns of movement. He may (unintentionally) try to compensate for the problems of abnormal postural tone by using abnormal patterns of movement to carry out daily activities of living as best he can. If these limited and inadequate patterns persist (which they usually do, as they can be relatively successful in enabling the child to achieve certain aims) he learns to use them as a basis for future movements, which may in turn become increasingly limited. It is essential that parents and people who work with children with cerebral palsy learn how to *handle* them as effectively as possible to enable them to move in a more normal and more efficient way.

A therapist can help the adult learn how to handle the child so as to normalize his muscle tone as much as possible. The most effective way to develop and improve one's own handling skills is to feel the child under the guidance of a physiotherapist or occupational therapist. It takes time and practice to become aware of slight changes in muscle tone. During their training, physiotherapists and occupational therapists spend many hours acquiring these skills. Speech and language therapists put similar emphasis on auditory training; that is, the ability to identify very slight changes in voice and speech production. An increasing, but as yet limited, number will have had further training which provides valuable experience in handling children. However, it is important to appreciate that changes in the child's muscle tone will vary, depending on who is handling him, the time of day and so on. By careful handling, the abnormal patterns of movement can be inhibited to varying degrees and more normal patterns of movement be facilitated. The way in which a child is fed, carried, dressed/undressed, bathed, changed, sat, stood and laid down are of vital importance. These situations become opportunities to help the child learn to move more easily and in a more normal way. Careful assessment and understanding of the child's difficulties and abilities are very important.

There are many forms of treatment in current usage. The Bobath Concept is an internationally recognized and respected approach which was devised and developed in England by the late Dr Karel and Mrs Berta Bobath. Therapists from different backgrounds work together to analyse *what* the child is and is not able to do. This leads on to further questions, such as *how* does the child achieve what he does and *why* is he unable to achieve other skills? Therapy aims to identify the child's *unique* needs, leading to an individualized therapy plan which will equip him with the skills required for functional activities such as sitting and eating.

An essential aspect of treatment is the continuous monitoring of how the child achieves success, as continued use of abnormal patterns can lead to later problems. The child's treatment aims to improve his functioning as he changes and develops. There is a great deal of emphasis on parent training since, as has already been explained, *everyday handling and management are part of treatment*. If a child is held so that he can see his parent's face, communication becomes easier. If his clothes are removed in a way that prevents him from pushing back and enables him to help himself, he will remain calmer, be easier to undress and learn more through the process.

Let us consider a possible mealtime situation for the child with cerebral palsy. He is sitting in a chair watching television. He is happy and relaxed and can maintain his balance well. The programme ends and the child hears food being prepared. The smells waft towards him; he is hungry and eager to eat. The telephone rings and his mother answers it. He becomes agitated by the sudden noise and movement. His muscle tone may increase. His mother replaces the telephone and brings in the meal. It is too hot to eat and the child becomes distressed. As he becomes more upset his body stiffens. He pushes back against the chair and his bottom slips forward. He tries to talk and the effort increases his muscle tone, his head moves back and his mouth opens very wide. His mother reassures him and tries to bring his head forward. However his body and legs are still stiff, his head is pressed against the chair back and his bottom is sliding down even further in the chair. If the child were to continue eating in an extended position he might well cough and risk food going 'down the wrong way'; that is, into the airway. As well as addressing the child's emotional needs, this adult must also be aware of how to handle her child so that she can help to reduce muscle tone, inhibit the abnormal pattern of extension (pushing back) and enable her child to move back into a more upright, symmetrical position and so on. It is only then that they *both* have the chance to continue the meal successfully.

The child's ability to eat and drink is dependent on his physical skills, especially head and trunk control. Good handling and seating are essential, for, without them, attempts at improving eating and drinking will be of limited value.

CHAPTER FIVE

◆ POSITIONING

◆

THE importance of good positioning for both communication and eating/drinking cannot be overemphasized (*see Chapters 3 and 4*). Whilst the child's physical needs have to be met, we must not forget the needs of the feeder; therefore when experimenting with seating do not overlook her comfort. No one benefits in the long term if the feeder is in pain or discomfort during the meal. Backache is a common problem in both parents and professionals. Making sure that the carer does not suffer is in the interests of both people. Individual differences in size and height of feeders should be taken into consideration when planning therapy. Remember that nearly all children should be *fed upright*. Only young babies are 'designed' to be fed in a reclining position (*see Chapter 2*).

Many children with cerebral palsy feel much happier on someone's lap and they may indeed benefit from the physical and emotional support that this provides. However, it is important to remember that as children grow they can become very manipulative, especially at mealtimes. It is therefore advisable to get the child used to a chair or prone stander or standing frame from as early an age as is felt appropriate by his physiotherapist or occupational therapist. The aim of positioning for

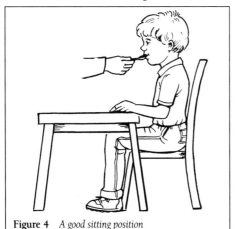

Figure 4   *A good sitting position*

mealtimes is to enable the child to be upright, in mid-line (symmetrical alignment) with an elongated back of neck. (See Figure 4.) It is not possible to describe specific positions best suited to children with particular problems, because no two children are the same. However, the following principles are very important and should be considered by all members of the team helping the child.

RELATIVE POSITION OF CHILD TO FEEDER

The height and position of the child who is eating in relation to the feeder is a crucial factor in ensuring that the mealtime is successful and safe.

◆ PRACTICAL EXERCISE 5

This is to allow you to experience the effect of the relative position of the feeder to the person being fed. You will need another person to help you with this exercise.

Firstly try just talking to each other and then take it in turns to feed each other, adopting the following positions (the feeder will be called 'A' and the person being fed 'B').

1   'A' higher than 'B'.
2   'A' behind 'B'.
3   'A' beside 'B'.
4   'A' opposite 'B'.

How did these different positions feel? Which position was the most uncomfortable — and why? Which was the most comfortable — and why?

29

Most people will have found that they preferred sitting opposite one another. Why should that be? This position has the important advantage of enabling you to see each other's faces easily. A successful mealtime depends on good communication and the two are inextricably linked. This face-to-face contact remains important when the child who is eating has a visual impairment. (However, sometimes totally blind children prefer to be side-by-side with their feeder.) It should therefore be no surprise that being able to establish eye contact is a priority. It is possible to do this while sitting next to each other as long as 'A' is at the appropriate height and turns her head towards 'B'. If the child tends to push into extension when he looks up, try to avoid sitting higher than him. *An extended head, neck and body position makes eating and drinking difficult, uncomfortable and potentially dangerous.*

PROXIMITY OF FOOD/UTENSILS AND SO ON

This may seem an obvious point, but it is worth checking that whatever will be needed is as conveniently placed as possible before starting the meal. If the carer has to get up during the meal this is distracting for the child. Having food, drink and utensils in view of the child helps him to anticipate his meal (although this might overexcite some children). Most children benefit from being able to touch their food, drink and utensils, so this proximity is essential for them.

NOISE LEVELS

Do not underestimate the effect of a noisy environment. It may be difficult for the child to concentrate on the meal and communicate with the carer if, for example, the radio, television and washing machine are on. Schools are faced with a particularly awkward situation as noise and activity levels at mealtimes tend to be very high. It only takes one dropped tray and a crying child to upset several other children. Where background music is played this only adds to the distraction, which is usually unhelpful to the children. (*See Chapter 12.*)

Creating small separate groups for eating in a quieter environment can help. Such a group could include children who can eat independently with those who are less skilled, and thereby encourage a more pleasant and beneficial social atmosphere. Being part of a frantic, noisy group will not help a child develop useful social skills. The effect of noise is particularly relevant where children have a visual or hearing impairment: they are more dependent on auditory cues, which are far harder to discriminate in a general hubbub.

VISUAL DISTRACTIONS

This problem was touched on in the previous section. However, I would like to highlight the often intrusive effect of television on communication at mealtimes. Whilst television can be a stimulating medium, it is not recommended as a mealtime companion. It is *no substitute for real two-way communication.* Many people find that television alters their style of conversation. Often, people will half-listen to what is said by those around them and continue to make eye contact with the screen. If television is specifically used as a distractor, do try to 'wean' the child from it as soon as possible.

Light sources themselves, such as sunshine or fluorescent lights shining onto faces or sunlight flickering through windows, particularly through venetian blinds, may cause discomfort.

SITTING OR STANDING?

It may seem strange to suggest that a child be fed while standing. Most children, once they start walking, will happily eat food that is accessible and, indeed, adults often eat when standing and walking. Many children with cerebral palsy have a standing frame or prone stander which may be useful at mealtimes, for the following reasons:

1 Standing tends to normalize muscle tone in response to the stimulation of being up against gravity.

2 When standing the child bears weight through the hips and feet, which provides some stability from which other movements can be made.

The above factors are most relevant to hypotonic (floppy) and athetoid children.

3 Standing is the position of most extension (straightening) of the body. It may therefore help to inhibit flexion (bending) in a child whose predominant pattern of movement is one of flexion.

4 Standing eases descent of food and fluid into the stomach.

5 Gravity facilitates the passing of stools, so that standing may be helpful for children who are constipated and may help to prevent reflux (where food returns from the stomach into the oesophagus (gullet)).

Standing is not suitable if it makes the child push back. Although straps may be required for good security and posture, care should be taken to avoid pressure on the abdomen (stomach), especially in a stander which is tilted forward (prone stander).

The importance of the advice of a physiotherapist or occupational therapist cannot be overemphasized. Careful observation and some trial and error sessions will be needed in order to ascertain what support is most helpful to the child. Each child has his own special requirements and will benefit from specific suggestions made. Do bear in mind that *mealtimes can be hard work for the child with cerebral palsy*.

Sitting

We may at times have unrealistic expectations and demand that the child do his best in all areas simultaneously. It is expecting a lot for a child to sit, chew and self-feed simultaneously. Remember that a baby has normally acquired head control before chewing develops

and has good sitting balance before self-feeding commences. We would not learn to play the flute while balancing on one leg! *Seating for mealtime postural stability may be different from seating designed to improve active sitting balance in therapy. When the child is developing chewing or self-feeding skills, he should not have to concentrate on balance at the same time.*

The following points are intended to be used as guidelines alongside discussion with the child's therapists, other staff and parents. Do experiment but please *allow reasonable time before giving up with seemingly unsuccessful approaches*.

Height of table in relation to height of chair

Classically, proportions allow the feet, knees and hips to be at right angles (90 degrees), the shoulders to be down (not hunched) and the elbows to be at nearly 90 degrees. (See Figure 5.) Some children, such as those that tend to slump, need the table to be higher. Others may go into extension if the table is too high.

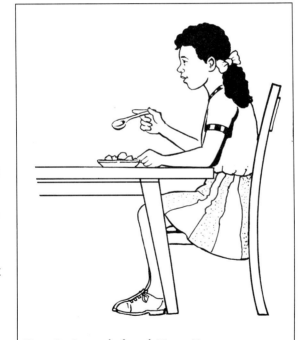

Figure 5 *An example of a good sitting position*
Note: Right angle at feet, knees and hips; bottom well back; shoulders are down; elbow at nearly 90 degrees; table at appropriate height and distance; good back support provided.

31

Height of seat

In general the height of the seat from the floor or foot-rest should be such that the child's knees and ankles are at right angles. The child should be at the same height as family members at mealtimes.

Distance between chair and table

The child should have a firm base for his forearms to rest on, to help keep his shoulders nicely rounded and his elbows slightly flexed. If the child is too close to the table, the pressure of his body against it may stimulate hyperextension (excessive pushing back and straightening of the body and limbs). It could adversely affect breathing and/or the passage of food into the stomach and could cause vomiting.

If the child is too far from the table, the slight touch of his hands on the table may stimulate rapid withdrawal of the arms.

Foot support

The child's feet should be supported on the floor or foot-rest to increase his stability. This may be particularly important for children with a visual impairment so that they feel safe and on a firm base. However, there are some children who are stimulated by pressure on the soles of the feet to go into extension. Such children may need to start off without a foot-rest.

Back of chair

The back of the chair should provide adequate support. A headrest may stimulate pushing back, especially if it is level with the back of the head. The chair should promote an upright head and body posture. The head should be in mid-line (symmetrical alignment) with an elongated back of the neck. Adaptions that can help to elongate the back of the child's neck, such as a rolled up towel, 'snake' or neck cushion (see Figures 6a, 6b, 6c) can be invaluable at mealtimes.

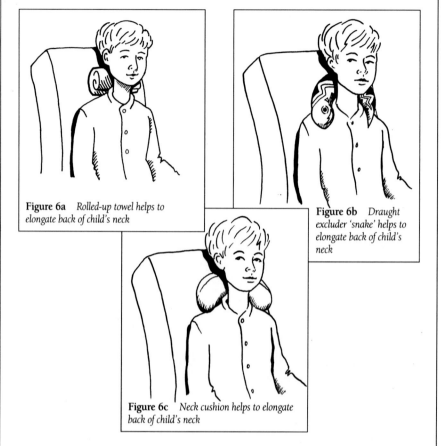

Figure 6a *Rolled-up towel helps to elongate back of child's neck*

Figure 6b *Draught excluder 'snake' helps to elongate back of child's neck*

Figure 6c *Neck cushion helps to elongate back of child's neck*

Hips

Remember that the hips should be at 90 degrees flexion. The child's bottom should be stable in the chair to provide better trunk and head control. The correct seat depth, angle of seat to back and thigh position are vital. A non-slip mat placed on the chair under the bottom can be helpful. A pelvic strap may be required to stabilize the child's hips.

Seating adaptions

If these are in use, do not forget to reassess their value regularly. As the child changes, so do his seating requirements. It is very easy to continue using adaptions long after they are needed, as when prolonging the use of a headrest after the child's head control has improved.

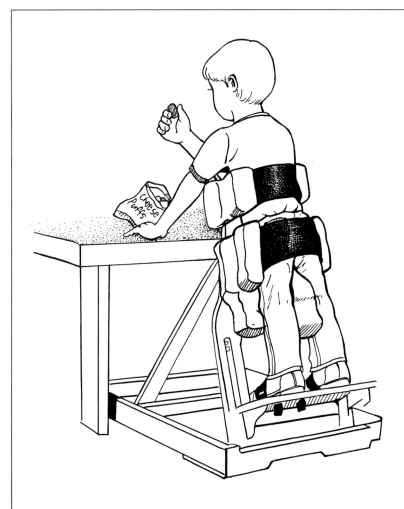

Figure 7   *Standing*
Note: Feet at right angles; good stabilization at hip, trunk and knees; left hand firmly on the table to provide stability; food near child.

Standing

The principles of relative heights and distances are the same as for sitting, although the hips and knees are obviously not at right angles (see Figure 7).

Feet

The child's feet should be stable and well supported to provide a good base. They should be flat, in a mid-position, with weight being taken evenly.

Hips

Aim for symmetry and alignment with the feet.

◆ SAFETY NOTES

---

1   During eating and drinking, maintaining elongation of the back of the child's neck is recommended for safety reasons.

2   Where a child is firmly strapped into his chair, standing frame or prone stander, the feeder should know how to unstrap the child should he choke and require prompt intervention.

3   When in a highchair, a child should always be secured with a safety harness which can be quickly released by the feeder if necessary. Do not leave the child unsupervised.

4   Note whether abnormal patterns of movement could tip the chair or stander. Make appropriate adjustments where necessary to prevent an accident occurring.

◆ REMEMBER

Time spent on careful and appropriate positioning is time well spent. Good positioning is the foundation for improving eating and drinking skills.

◆

CHAPTER SIX

ASSESSMENT

◆

THE TEAM

It may be extremely difficult to assess a routine activity such as eating that is often taken for granted. A range of people may be involved in helping a child with cerebral palsy improve his eating and drinking. These people, who together form 'the team', may include the following.

The child's parents, and possibly other family members, such as grandparents, brothers, sisters

These are the most important people in the team. In particular an older child or young adult is a very important part of the team and should be involved in making decisions. His consent and co-operation are essential in, for example, controlling dribbling and helping him to eat independently. Respite carers should also be involved in the management of their residents.

Doctors

Paediatricians (who specialize in treating children) and/or general practitioners usually have overall responsibility for the child's medical management and are able to refer to staff such as therapists, dieticians and other doctors for further help as appropriate.

Nurses

Where children are in hospital, nurses will play an important part in their daily care. Community nurses, general practice nurses, school nurses and health visitors may be involved in the child's care. Specialist nurses may be able to advise on specific areas, such as management of tube-feeding, where required.

Speech and language therapists

These therapists can advise on non-verbal communication, language, play, speech and voice production. In addition, some offer specialist help with eating, drinking and dribbling problems.

Physiotherapists

Physiotherapists specialize in movement. They can advise on how best to carry the child, and help develop better movement skills leading on to greater mobility and function. They monitor possible problems such as hip dislocation and scoliosis (spinal curvature) and work with orthopaedic surgeons. In conjunction with other therapists they may be able to offer very useful advice on positioning at mealtimes. They may be involved in the provision of equipment, such as seats, standing frames and shoes. Physiotherapists can also advise on chest care where this is appropriate.

Occupational therapists

Occupational therapists specialize in activities of daily living (ADL), such as dressing, bathing, toilet training and self-feeding. They are also interested in visual perception (making sense of what we see), eye–hand co-ordination and play. In addition, they may recommend the use of specialized cutlery, chairs or standing frames and sometimes help with providing them. They can advise on possible house alterations, such as the provision of ramps.

There are areas of common knowledge as well as specializations between therapists and not all children need to be seen by all three kinds of therapist. A specific therapist may be the 'key' worker at different times in the child's life. Discussion of the child's needs should establish what input is required. The main focus is to *equip the parents* with the skills appropriate to *their* child, as they deal with the daily situations of mealtimes, dressing and washing.

Educational staff

Teachers, nursery nurses and support staff look at the child's eating and drinking in the context of the school day. In some areas, pre-school teachers provide a home-based programme. In such cases it is imperative that they discuss their advice with the child's therapists to ensure maximum benefit. Specialist teachers such as teachers of children with visual or hearing impairments may also be involved where appropriate.

Dieticians

Dieticians specialize in nutrition. They are able to analyse information on food and liquid intake and can recommend supplements if appropriate. They can also advise on specific problems such as constipation, allergies, tube-feeding and special diets for people with conditions such as diabetes.

Dental surgeons

The child with cerebral palsy should have regular dental check-ups from the age of approximately two and a half years in the same way as any other young child. In some areas there are particular dentists who have experience of seeing children with special needs.

Psychologists

Psychologists specialize in learning and behaviour. As mealtime behaviour problems are very common, a psychologist may be able

to contribute to advice on management through discussion with parents and other adults as well as through contact with the child.

Psychiatrists

These are doctors with specialist knowledge of emotion, behaviour and personality disorders. They are able to offer counselling to individuals as well as the family as a whole.

Social workers

Practical help, such as arranging respite care and informing parents of benefits to which they are entitled, is provided by social workers. They may also offer counselling services.

Audiologists

Audiologists are able to assess children's hearing. This is particularly important for children with cerebral palsy where screening tests may not have identified a hearing loss. 'Sense' staff may also be able to offer developmental assessment and advice. (*See Appendix IV.*)

Ophthalmologists

Ophthalmologists are able to assess children's vision. This is particularly important for children with cerebral palsy where screening tests may not have identified a visual impairment. 'Sense' staff may also be able to offer developmental assessment and advice. (*See Appendix IV.*)

Orthopaedic surgeons

These are doctors specializing in bones and joints. They monitor the position and mobility of joints such as the hips, knees, ankles and spine.

Orthotists

Orthotists are specialists in providing aids, such as splints and braces, which affect positioning.

ENT surgeons

These are doctors specializing in disorders of the ears, nose and throat.

Plastic surgeons

Plastic surgeons are doctors who deal with structural deformity. This may be present from birth, such as cleft lip and palate, or acquired following trauma, such as a road traffic accident.

Radiologists

These are doctors who interpret X-rays, Barium swallows and videofluoroscopy (see page 50).

Radiographers

Radiographers are the staff who take X-rays, or perform Barium swallows and videofluoroscopy (see page 50).

Gastroenterologists

These doctors specialise in disorders of the digestive system.

It is clear that many people may be involved in helping a child who has difficulty with eating and drinking. The wealth of information coming from different sources may be confusing for parents. Some areas have therefore adopted a 'key worker' scheme. This 'key' person is responsible for ensuring good liaison with the family and may be approached where clarification is required, or when problems arise.

ASSESSMENT CONSIDERATIONS

Mealtimes involve many interrelated factors which need to be assessed both independently and interactively. However, for clarity, I have considered them as follows.

Age and developmental level of the child

As the development of eating and drinking follows a sequential pattern, a child's age tells us what we might expect him to be able to do. However, some children may not be able to eat or drink as expected for their age. There may be a similar delay in the development of other skill areas. It is nevertheless important to provide a range of experiences that can stimulate progress. Children often display a scattered range of abilities and with appropriate help many mealtime skills can be achieved and enjoyed by the children, their families and carers.

Previous feeding experiences
Method of feeding

Children's early feeding experiences are of very great importance and often help adults to understand the presenting difficulties. For example, it is common for babies with cerebral palsy to be fed via a nasogastric tube. This involves the (often frequent) passing of a thin catheter (tube) through one nostril down into the stomach. This restricts the nasal airway and may be very uncomfortable. In addition, the baby may require suctioning if he is unable to keep his mouth, throat and chest clear of secretions. The baby's early experiences of stimulation to the mouth may therefore be associated with discomfort, fear and even pain. *Some babies may have been force-fed, so that they fear the whole feeding experience.* The baby may also be unable to explore by putting his hands, feet or toys to his mouth.

It is easy to see how the baby can quickly become hypersensitive (react negatively) to any stimulation in the mouth or around the face. There may also be additional problems, such as 'tactile defensiveness'. (*See Chapter 7 for more details.*)

Variety of food

If a child has difficulty eating, he may only be given foods or liquids which are known to be taken satisfactorily. If attempts at changing the diet are unsuccessful the feeder may decide to continue feeding as before. In the long run this may make the development of, for example, chewing far more difficult as the child and feeder become accustomed to a limited range of tastes, textures and temperatures. The longer the child's intake is restricted in this way the more difficult it is likely to be to effect change. In addition his diet may become deficient in certain nutrients.

Feeder

The child may have been in a hospital where frequent staff changes have prevented the establishment of a trusting feeding relationship. On the other hand, a child may have only been fed by one person (usually the mother) and may refuse to be fed by anyone else. It is important to find out how the child's eating and drinking vary with different feeders. The feeder's attitude to food and drink may be relevant. For example, she may strongly dislike some of the foods that she is giving to the child. The feeder's attitude and sensitivity to the child's needs should also be considered.

Previous positions used

The child may have become used to being fed passively on someone's lap or being sat in front of a favourite video. Such habits need to be discussed and ideas pooled in order to alter the situation to enable the child to eat more independently, using more mature movement patterns.

Medical aspects and safety issues

There may be specific problems such as reflux (regurgitation) and vomiting which affect feeding. These need to be assessed and discussed fully, with appropriate action being taken if necessary. Eating and drinking can present hazards. Concerns regarding safety are discussed in Chapter 7.

Current position

It is imperative to seek help from the child's physiotherapist and occupational therapist. As discussed in Chapters 4 and 5, good positioning is fundamental to successful mealtimes. It is important to ask the following: **What position is used — and why?** and **What support is required — and why?** Seating needs to be regularly reviewed as the child's growth and changing condition require a flexible approach. A headrest that was helpful at one stage may be unnecessary a few months later. The height of the tray will need altering as the child grows taller. It is particularly important to aim for symmetry, and alignment of head and trunk. Most importantly, the head should be upright, the back of the neck elongated and the chin slightly tucked in, as shown in Figure 5. (*See Chapter 5 for details.*)

It is important to note how the child is positioned or moved following a meal as this may affect digestion. Some children are less likely to retain air (wind), or be constipated, or vomit, or have reflux problems if they are stood up after meals.

Texture of food/consistency of drink

The texture of food and consistency of drink offered to the child should be considered.

Texture of food

It is difficult to describe textures accurately. Consider the variety of adjectives which can be applied to food texture: smooth, lumpy, dry, runny, stringy, chewy, soggy, mashed, chopped, diced, crunchy, sticky, slippery. As many of these terms are easily misinterpreted it is helpful if those people who feed the child jointly assess the texture of the food given to the child. Knowing what textures the child is used to helps adults to understand what opportunities the child has to suck, bite and chew.

It is important to know *how* the child copes with different textures; for example, he may suck yogurt but chew a biscuit. It is essential to be aware of any difficulties that the child experiences with particular foods so that they may be avoided; for example, he may choke on sausages or peas. The way in which he deals with single or combined textures should be noted. For example, he may be able to chew cake as long as it is not mixed with custard. Combining these two foods may lead to sucking. It is also important to remember that some foods change in texture after a few seconds or minutes. Consider how cereals alter as they absorb milk.

It is worth spending time analysing food textures and their effect on the child's eating as this information will be helpful in planning future food preparation and presentation.

Consistency of drink

Drinks, like food, vary in their consistency, although the possibilities are more limited. We tend to think of two broad categories, thin and thick. Most liquids, such as milk and water, are thin. Thick drinks such as milkshakes are less common although, as long as they are *smooth*, thick liquids are often easier for children to drink than thinner liquids. It is important to establish what the child likes and how his drinking skills vary depending on the consistency of the liquid offered.

Speed of feeding

Do be aware of the *rate* at which the child is given food and drink and consider how it affects his ability to cope. For example, too fast a rate may cause the child to choke. Altering the rate at which a meal is given may be very beneficial to the child.

◆ PRACTICAL EXERCISE 6

This is to highlight how the rate at which a person is fed affects his ability to eat and drink. You will need a partner for this exercise.

Select two textures of food such as yogurt and some biscuits and a glass of water. Take it in turns to feed each other as *quickly* as possible.

How does it feel to be given food that you are not ready to eat? It is probably unpleasant and perhaps alarming.

Now hold the drink to your partner's mouth and give her a drink as *slowly* as possible.

How does it feel to anticipate drinking when the liquid does not flow as expected? It is probably frustrating.

Continuity of approach

It is important to establish how much opportunity the child has had to get used to any new ideas, whether these involve a different utensil, texture, room, feeder or other variables. New ideas may not have worked because they were not tried out for long enough.

Communication

As discussed in Chapter 3, it is important to develop the child's ability to communicate at mealtimes. Some specific questions to address are:

1 Does the position the child is in allow for face-to-face contact, use of picture charts and so on?

2. Is the child given the opportunity to make choices, such as refusing food or requesting more?

3. How does the child indicate the above?

4. Are the child's choices respected?

5. Does everyone who feeds the child know how the child expresses himself? Sign language, gesture, eye pointing and so on may all be used.

6. If the child has a picture/symbol chart, is it *available at mealtimes*?

7. Are the pictures/symbols *required at mealtimes* on the chart?

It is also important to encourage communication between children by placing them appropriately in relation to each other. Where a child has additional problems, such as impaired vision and/or hearing, specific considerations must be given to ensure that the room is adequately lit and that extraneous noise is limited. (*See Chapters 3 and 11 for more details.*)

Breathing pattern

Note how the child's breathing pattern changes before, during and after meals. In particular note how the child's breathing rate/depth is likely to change before, during or following drinking or eating. Look and listen for changes. Does the child's breathing become noisy following a drink? Does the child cough when drinking? The child may need more frequent and longer pauses during drinking to enable breathing to return to a more normal pattern. **If there is any concern regarding the child's ability to eat or drink safely seek medical advice.**

Oral–motor (mouth movement)

Careful observation is important in planning therapy. The following is intended to highlight some common difficulties.

Head position

When considering mouth movement it is essential to look at the head and trunk position, as this will influence oral–motor functioning.

◆ PRACTICAL EXERCISE 7

This is to highlight the importance of good positioning for safety reasons.

Imagine that you are giving 'the kiss of life' (mouth-to-mouth resuscitation) to someone. How do you position the head? You tip it back and open the mouth fully so that the airway (windpipe) is wide open for maximum airflow.

We therefore want a different head position when the aim is to *prevent* food and drink from entering the airway, to help the child swallow safely. We all normally swallow with the back of our neck elongated and our chin slightly tucked in. This is the position in which the *airway is most protected*.

Look at the child's head position. Is it upright, forward or tipped back? Is it in mid-line or to one side? It may vary depending on factors such as muscle tone, level of activity, visual and auditory distractions such as television, mobiles hanging from a ceiling and relative position of the feeder. For example, if the feeder is seated higher than the child, this could lead to the child tipping back his head in order to see the feeder's face. With the help of a physiotherapist or occupational therapist assess how to achieve a better head position in order to enable the child to eat and drink more efficiently and safely.

Jaw movement

As we saw in Chapter 2, the young baby's mouth opens wide when feeding. It is only after the development of head control that the jaw starts to move less; that is, it has become more stable, and opens just the right amount to take in food or drink.

This is to help you experience the importance of jaw stability for eating or drinking.

Try drinking some water or eating a biscuit while opening and closing your mouth. You will see how difficult, if not impossible, it is to use your lips and tongue to control the food or drink while your jaw moves up and down.

Look at the child's jaw both at rest and at mealtimes and note the degree of movement used. It may be very difficult for the child to open his mouth, particularly so in the child who tends to be flexed (bent).

These children may also tend to bite strongly on the spoon (bite reflex — this is discussed in Chapter 7). The child may open his mouth too wide, which can lead to a pattern of extension (pushing back). In the hypotonic (floppy) child, the jaw may be lax and open. The child's jaw may open and close repeatedly at the sight of food or after food has been swallowed. Should these sorts of problems occur it may be necessary to provide extra support to the head and/or back of neck and/or jaw to provide the stability required. Where there is excessive flexion, the physiotherapist or occupational therapist can help by advising on how to handle and position the child in such a way as to provide greater extension and thus help to provide a more normal combination of flexion and extension.

Where there is too much extension, advice on handling and position can help to inhibit this pattern of movement and provide a more normal combination of flexion and extension.

Lip movement

Many hypotonic (floppy) children often have difficulty controlling their lips and frequently breathe through their mouth. A spastic (stiff) child may have difficulty parting the lips and may have a top lip which is pulled back and slightly upward (retracted). Athetoid children may have involuntary facial movements and grimacing.

When assessing lip movement it is important to consider how the way in which the child is fed may affect lip activity. For example, if food is scraped off against the top teeth the child does not have the opportunity to use his top lip to remove food from the spoon. Feeding too quickly may increase involuntary movement. It can also stimulate retraction (pulling up) of the upper lip, which is due to spasticity (increased tone).

Tongue movement

Many children with cerebral palsy use an immature sucking pattern characterized by rhythmical forward–backward tongue movement and vertical jaw movement. However, many of them have a tongue thrust which is different, in that it is part of a pattern of extension; that is, it occurs more when the child's head and trunk are extended. There is an increase in muscle tone which makes the tongue appear bunched. It does *not* move rhythmically and may protrude out of the mouth. Tongue thrust is described more fully in Chapter 7.

The jaw may open widely in association with tongue movements. Both immature sucking and tongue thrust may be seen in the same child. It is helpful to note whether the tongue can move to one side of the mouth more easily than to the other. Children may have difficulty in propelling food to the back of the mouth to swallow because of limited tongue movement.

Cheeks

It is difficult to appreciate how our cheeks are involved in eating and drinking. It is most obvious in babies, where fatty tissue called 'sucking pads' assists in sucking. The cheeks provide stability and enable us to store food in our mouth. Children with cerebral palsy may have poor control of their cheeks. If food becomes lodged in his cheeks the child may require help to clear them.

Sensory aspects

Touch

The child's reaction to being touched, moved and so on should be considered, as it will affect the way in which people should handle him. Some children do not appear to respond to touch, while others move away from any tactile (touch) stimulation.

Some children seem unaware of certain sensations; for example, a child may not realize that he is dribbling because his chin does not feel wet or because the way it feels seems natural to him. Some children will enjoy touching food, while others will dislike it.

The sensation of clothing touching the child may interfere with mealtimes, for instance if the bib used is too tight around the child's neck or is made of an irritating fabric. The texture of the carer's clothes should also be considered — a mohair sweater may irritate the child, for example.

Visual and auditory stimuli

It is important to note how the child responds to his surroundings both by *sight* and by *sound*. Some children have great difficulty in tolerating a highly stimulating environment.

Smell

Assessing how the child reacts to different smells is helpful. Smells may stimulate mouth movement and can be helpful therapeutically.

Temperature

The child's reaction to different temperatures of food and drink should also be considered. Many children prefer warm food and some show a dislike of very cold food and drink.

Taste

Assessing the child's reaction to different tastes is also helpful. Many children will have experienced only a limited range of tastes.

Utensils — see Appendix I

The child may use any one or a combination of the following: bottle, cup, straw, spoon, fork, knife, bowls, plates, and, of course, fingers. It is important not only to note the properties of the utensil, such as the material it is made of, its shape, size, colour and weight, but also to analyse *how* it is used. When trying out a new utensil, it is important to allow sufficient time for the child to become used to it before abandoning its use in favour of an alternative. Where a child has been given a long time to try out a new item or management idea without success, do analyse the situation to establish why the approach has been unsuccessful so that a different approach can be instigated. Some examples are given below.

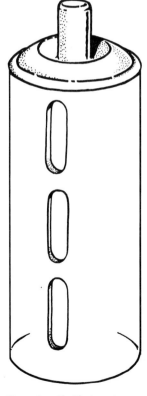

Bottle

◆ **Size and shape:** affects ease of use by feeder and child. Affects ease with which it can be cleaned.
◆ **Coloured/clear:** affects ability of feeder and child to see contents.
◆ **Special design:**
   the Playtex System (see Figure 8a). Comprises a plastic holder to which is attached a disposable plastic feeding bag which shrinks as the liquid is drunk, thus reducing air intake.

Figure 8a *The Playtex system*

the Haberman feeder (see Figure 8b). This bottle's design enables the feeder to alter the rate and ease with which the liquid flows.

the Rosti bottle (see Figure 8c). Can be squeezed to aid liquid flow.

MagMag system (see Figure 8d). Has interchangeable lids, including a rubber spout which may be useful if a child is unable to suck from a conventional teat.

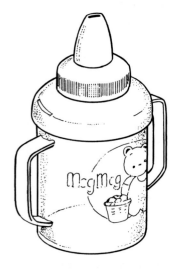

Figure 8d   MagMag cup with spout attachment

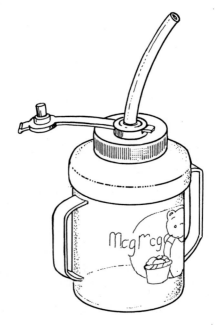

Figure 8e   MagMag cup with straw insert

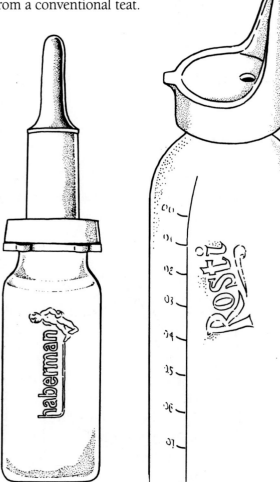

Figure 8b   The Haberman feeder   **Figure 8c**   The Rosti bottle

Teat

◆ **Size:** too large a teat for the size of the child's mouth might cause gagging.

◆ **Length:** too long a teat for the size of the child's mouth might cause gagging.

◆ **Width:** too wide a teat may lead to excessive mouth opening. Too narrow a teat may make lip seal too difficult to accomplish.

◆ **Shape:** needs to be appropriate to the shape of the child's mouth.

◆ **Firmness/softness:** a child may tire sucking on a hard teat. If the teat is too soft it may not provide the mouth with adequate stimulation to produce sucking. For some children a soft teat may lead to a too rapid rate of flow.

◆ **Number and size of holes:** note any additional enlargement that has been made.

- **Rate of flow:** assess whether this is appropriate for the child; for example, excessive rate of flow may result in the child spluttering.
- **Anti-colic mechanism:** as built into the Haberman feeder.

Remember that some of these properties, notably firmness, will change with use.

- **How the teat is used/manner of presentation:** consider the following:
    - How the child is held.
    - The position of the child's head.
    - The angle at which the bottle is held.
    - How far into the mouth the teat extends.
    - The speed with which it is put into and removed from the child's mouth.
    - How frequently it is removed.
    - Changes noticed within a feed, such as sucking rate slowing as the feed progresses.
    - Liquid loss.
    - Time taken.
    - Amount taken.
    - Any tendency to splutter.

Cup

- **Size:** appropriateness for child.
- **Material:** how it feels in the mouth, safety considerations.
- **Hardness/softness:** a softer cup can be squeezed to form a spout.
- **Thickness/thinness:** how it feels in the mouth.
- **Coloured/clear:** the latter enables the child/feeder to see the liquid.
- **Straight or flared rim:** a flared rim can provide a useful 'resting' point for a child's lower lip.

- **Aperture:** wide/narrow rim; straight/slanted rim — the angled rim of the *Doidy* and *Cheyne* cups facilitates drinking (see Figures 9a and 9b).

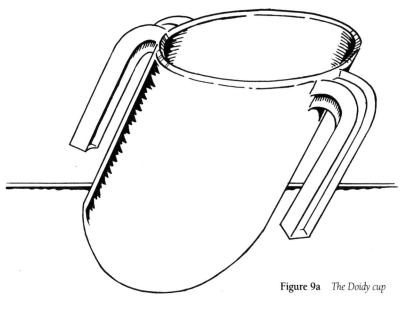

Figure 9a *The Doidy cup*

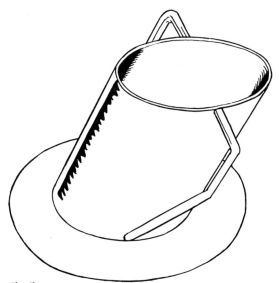

Figure 9b *The Cheyne cup*

- ◆ **Training lids:** the spouts often encourage biting and/or sucking in children with drinking difficulties.
- ◆ **Insert lids** such as Púr, MagMag and Cheyne (see Figures 9c, 9d and 9e); the holes provide a helpful means of controlling liquid flow.

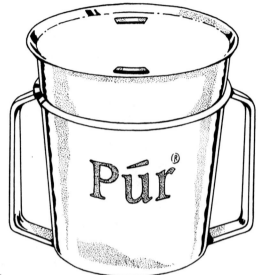

Figure 9c   *The Púr cup*
Note: The cup has two slits.

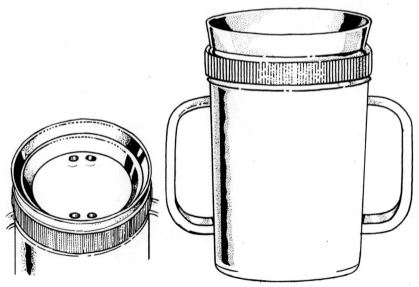

Figure 9d   *The MagMag cup*
Note: The cup has two medium-sized holes.

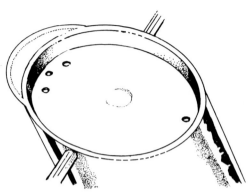

Figure 9e   *Cheyne cup with insert lid*

- ◆ **Presence/number of handles:** note their size, shape, position and ease of use for child/feeder as appropriate. Seek advice from a physiotherapist or occupational therapist regarding independent drinking.
- ◆ **Weighted base:** provides stability.
- ◆ **Insulated:** keep drinks warm/cool.
- ◆ **How the cup is used/manner of presentation:** consider the following.

  Position of child's head.
  Angle at which cup is held.
  Where the rim is placed.
  The speed with which the cup is put to/removed from the mouth.
  The speed at which liquid is given.
  How frequently the cup is removed.
  Any tendency to splutter.

Advice from a physiotherapist, speech and language therapist or occupational therapist should be sought where a child has difficulty co-ordinating breathing with eating and drinking.

Spoon

Properties of handle

◆ **Material:** some plastics are brittle and may break.

◆ **Size, Shape, Length, Weight, Angle:** all relevant to self-feeding — seek advice from a physiotherapist or occupational therapist.

Properties of bowl of spoon

◆ **Size:** should be appropriate for the size of the child's mouth; too large a spoon may cause discomfort and gagging.

◆ **Shape:** should be appropriate for the size of the child's mouth.

◆ **Material:** metal can feel cold and hard, but is strong; it may be difficult to remove food from a latex-covered spoon; should be strong enough to withstand a hard bite if the child has a bite reflex (this is discussed further in Chapter 7).

◆ **Depth:** it is easier to remove food from a shallow than from a deep-bowled spoon.

◆ **How item is used/manner of presentation:** consider the following.

  Angle from which it approaches — if it approaches from high up, the child may go into extension as a result of looking up to it; if it approaches from the side to which the child habitually turns, this will only serve to encourage this tendency.

  Amount of food — consider how much of the 'spoonful' is put/taken into the child's mouth each time. Remember that we often remove just some of the food from the spoon when feeding ourselves. Too much food may restrict tongue movement and cause gagging. Too little food may not provide enough stimulation or may be difficult to position in the mouth for chewing and swallowing.

  Where food is on the bowl of the spoon — it is easier to remove food from the end of the spoon.

  Speed: how quickly/slowly is the spoon put into/removed from the mouth? Remember that the child with cerebral palsy requires *time to adapt to changes*, including a spoon entering/leaving the mouth.

  How active is the child? Does the child have the *opportunity* to use his lips to remove food from the spoon? Is the food scraped off the child's upper gum/teeth? Is food tipped onto the child's tongue?

◆ PRACTICAL EXERCISE 9

This is to help you experience how the quantity of food in the mouth affects oral movement. You will need: (a) a carton of yogurt or similar, (b) two biscuits, such as 'digestives', (c) a few raisins, and (d) a paper towel or similar.

Compare the following:

1 Eat one teaspoon of yogurt, then one tablespoon of yogurt.

2 Take one bite of biscuit, then try to eat the rest *in one go*.

3 Eat one raisin, then eat several *squashed together*.

You will probably discover that too much food restricts tongue movement, whilst a very small amount, that is one raisin, requires very specific, complex tongue movements.

Feeder, or assistant where the child has some independence

Is the child fed by one or several people?

It is also worth considering how the feeder or assistant feels about the child she is feeding *and* about food in general terms. We all experience feelings of like, dislike and indifference towards people at times. We may also have strong feelings about certain foods, which might influence our attitude at mealtimes: for example, it could be difficult feeding something we strongly dislike to someone without conveying that fact!

This is to help you consider the importance of continuity of feeders.

Imagine that from now on you will never eat a meal with the same person for more than a couple of days. You will not know who you are going to sit with from one day to the next. Indeed, you may even find that your dining partner changes between courses! Whilst some variety is enjoyable, most of us would feel the above scenario undesirable. *The continuity of feeder* is particularly important where a child requires a lot of help. It enables a feeling of *trust and understanding* to develop, both of which are essential to the acquisition of improved mealtime skills.

Environment

The effect of the child's surroundings cannot be overemphasized.

◆ **PRACTICAL EXERCISE 11**

This is to help you focus on the effect that our surroundings have on us at mealtimes.

Imagine you are in an unfamiliar house. It is cold and your chair is uncomfortable. The table is wobbly. It is getting dark outside but no one has put on the light. The next-door neighbour is banging a nail into the shared wall or there is music on in an upstairs room and the television is on downstairs. You are now presented with a meal by an unfamiliar person. How do you feel? I expect that, even if the meal looked wonderful, it would be virtually impossible even for an adult to enjoy it under such circumstances. We need to consider *the effects of such stimuli as noise and lighting on children at mealtimes.*

Noise

What noises occur at mealtimes? They might include other children shouting or crying, a television and/or radio, microwave beeps, a washing machine running and outdoor sounds such as traffic. These stimuli can make it extremely difficult for a child to remain calm. Sudden noises may cause startled reactions and fear, leading to stiffening or an increase in involuntary movements. The child may be unable to pick out meaningful sounds such as voices amidst the general hubbub. This is particularly relevant when considering the child with a visual or hearing impairment, or a child with a learning disability.

Lighting

Is the room well lit? Lighting needs to be adequate but care should be taken to ensure that bright lights or the sun do not shine into children's eyes. Where a child has a visual impairment, care should be taken to ensure optimal lighting so that the child can see who is feeding him. Can he see the approaching food or drink, or does he need to be told what is being offered?

Level of activity

Are there lots of activities going on? At home these could be other children rushing about. In school there may be many people moving around, carrying trays, pushing trolleys and so on. For many children this makes focusing on their meal very difficult.

Time

How long is spent feeding the child? Mealtimes are often lengthy and can become tedious for both child and feeder. Consider how much food or drink is consumed within the first half of a meal compared to the second part. Measure this in millilitres or spoonfuls. You might wish to analyse the relative rate of eating throughout a meal in more detail. Remember that, if eating takes nearly two hours to complete, there will not be enough time between meals to enable the child to feel hungry.

Nutrition

When a child is very difficult to feed, the emphasis may be focused on merely getting food and liquid into the child, without necessarily considering the way the child is eating or drinking or his specific nutritional requirements.

Fluid intake may not be evaluated realistically if drinking is very difficult. Constipation is common and can be a major problem in children with cerebral palsy; this in turn can affect appetite. Inadequate fluid intake is often a contributory factor. When assessing a child's intake of both food and drink, do consider the following:

1 How often is the child offered food or drink?
2 Can the child request food or drink outside regular snack/mealtimes?
3 What type of food or drink is offered? Remember that variety can be provided in taste, texture, appearance and smell and it is very important to be aware of the child's reactions to these variations.
4 How much of the food or drink is taken at the beginning of the meal: that is, in the first 20 minutes?
5 How much of the food or drink is spilled, spat out or left on the bib?
6 What supplements, such as vitamins, and drugs, such as laxatives, are given?

Where possible, the advice of a dietician should be sought. Dieticians are specialists in nutrition and are able to assess a child's diet accurately and offer suggestions regarding such matters as increasing calorie and fluid intake. Unfortunately, dieticians are not always available; the information in Chapter 8 should provide some help.

Dental hygiene

Some children with cerebral palsy find it difficult to tolerate having their teeth cleaned. It is nonetheless important to consider what dental care is possible. The frequency and method of tooth cleaning should be considered. Factors such as the size and shape of the toothbrush head are important. The softness/hardness of the bristles should be considered. If the child swallows the toothpaste it is important to know whether or not it contains fluoride. The child's head position during tooth cleaning should be assessed. The state of the gums is very important as they provide the foundation for healthy teeth. Overgrown, puffy or bleeding gums should be noted. The number and condition of the teeth is important. Contact with a dentist should be made when the child is two and a half to three years of age. Further information can be found in Chapter 9.

Dribbling

Note how this is affected by changes in position, level of concentration, stress, emotion, activity, eating and drinking. Consider the child's sensory awareness — does he realize that he is dribbling? Also note whether the saliva tends to fall from one side of the mouth more than the other. See Chapter10 for further information.

Behaviour

Are mealtimes happy or are they seen as battlegrounds? Children are adept at picking up the emotions of adults and it is important for the feeders themselves to think about how they feel about the mealtime situation. Children who may be otherwise unable to assert themselves will often use mealtimes for this purpose.

Food refusal and fussiness generally gain adult attention. It is often very difficult to distinguish manipulative behaviour from the physical difficulty of eating, and careful assessment is required. For example, a child may gag deliberately to express dislike of a food and not because he is unable to eat it. The child's behaviour needs to be analysed. The child's reactions to different situations and people should be noted, as they may provide a key to improving mealtime behaviour.

Emotional factors

Feeding a child can be a highly emotional experience. It is important to be aware of the feelings of both the child and his feeder. A wide range of emotions, ranging from pleasure at a child's success to despair at apparent failure, is to be expected. Feelings are likely to change as the child grows older. Strong emotions of anger and guilt may be expressed. The child himself may need to express feelings of frustration, resentment and so on. This is important and he needs to know that his emotions have been acknowledged.

People working with the child and his family need to be aware of the psychological implications of feeding a child with special needs. They need to listen to the family and try to help them deal with their situation as successfully as possible.

Social, cultural and religious factors

It is important to remember that people do not always have the same ideas about eating and drinking. The advice of well intentioned family, friends and neighbours may conflict with professional guidelines, leading to additional confusion for the parents. Although 'family mealtimes' may not be the norm in some families, eating in a social context is often of great benefit to children with cerebral palsy.

Some cultures regard fat babies as being healthy, whereas others urge parents not to overindulge their offspring. In some religions the eating of certain foods is prohibited, so appropriate alternatives will need to be found. In many cultures it is common for children to be breast-fed for several years. A bottle may also be used until school age. Utensils may not be routinely used. Where hand-feeding is common practice we should be aware of the rules governing this tradition — the left hand may not be used for feeding. This has implications for the child who is unable to use his right hand because of physical disability. Seating may not be used routinely, which has implications for the child who is unable to support himself upright. Members of the extended family may hold an important position within the household and should therefore be involved in decision making.

◆ SUMMARY

I have highlighted the main areas to be assessed. Throughout any meal we should remember that eating and drinking involve much more than a mouth and the digestive system. Try to observe the child and feeder/assistant as a unit.

If you are the feeder and have the use of a video-recorder you might consider recording the mealtime to look at later. (I would not suggest that the child looks at it, unless he wishes to do so — our aim is to help the child, and not to upset him.) When noting different features, remember to ask yourself: What can the child do and how does he do it? What can't the child do and why can't he do it? This approach helps to establish the underlying causes of presenting problems which can be managed in therapy. Unless this occurs, inappropriate intervention may be undertaken. It is also important to note how the child *varies* in his eating or drinking. For example, what are the optimum circumstances for meals — with a particular feeder, a specific time of day, or when eating a favourite food? This information is important as new ideas should be implemented in situations which are most likely to promote success.

Where therapists are involved, it is important that they try to feed the children themselves, as pure observation cannot provide the information that can only be felt by 'hands on' experience. For example, a child may start to push back on seeing food approach. This may not be apparent to an observer, but is easily felt by someone holding him.

It is important to discuss the assessment together so that parents and therapists and school staff can agree a programme that will provide continuity. This is the most effective way of enabling the child to gain as much as possible from the whole mealtime experience. Remember to ask yourself: WHOSE MEAL IS IT?

CHAPTER SEVEN

MANAGEMENT OF EATING & DRINKING DIFFICULTIES

PRIORITIES

Preparation

The anticipation of meals involves stimulation of the senses such as smell and touch, emotions such as excitement and apprehension and has physical effects, for example the production of saliva.

It is important to prepare the child physically and emotionally to provide as calm an environment as possible, in order to help him to cope with these experiences.

Positioning

As described in Chapter 5, the child's position is fundamental to the quality of his eating and drinking skills. Advice on positioning should be sought from the therapy team. In general he should be in an upright position with his head in alignment with his body. His head should be in mid-line (symmetrical alignment) with an elongated back of neck so that the head is upright and the chin is slightly tucked in. (See Figure 5.)

Special seating may not be available when eating outside the home or school but, as long as the feeder or assistant is aware of the child's needs, it is often possible to adapt chairs using such items as rolled up towels, cushions and draught-excluder 'snakes' or similar. (See Figures 6a–c.) Remember that variation in the height and size of the feeder should be considered when suggesting positioning. Both the child and the feeder need to be comfortable.

Refer to Chapter 5 for further information on positioning.

Communication

Do provide as many opportunities as possible for the child to express hunger or thirst, food and drink preferences, choosing between food and drink, the wish to stop eating or drinking and so on. If the child uses a communication system such as pictures, line drawing pictograms eg. Rebuses and Makaton symbols or the more complex Blissymbolics do ensure that the pictures/symbols are accessible before and during mealtimes and, more importantly, that they are then used! Refer to Chapter 3 for further information on communication.

Nutrition

Children require a range of foods and drinks in order to thrive. It may seem that mealtimes are by necessity the time when the child *has* to be fed in *any way* just to meet these requirements. Parents and other adults may have felt obliged to push food or drink into a child who does not want it. Thus many children may have been 'force-fed' by their carers. Such experiences are counter-productive. Children may be force-fed because their carers are desperate for them to take food or drink and to be well nourished. Where this situation has occurred, it is essential to tackle it with the back-up of a team who can pool ideas and suggest alternative management strategies.

Refer to Chapter 8 for further information on nutrition.

Safety

Good positioning, as described in Chapter 5, enables the child to eat and drink more efficiently and safely. Children should never be left alone during a meal. The cough reflex was described in Chapter 2. It is vital in protecting the airway. Some children with cerebral palsy have an absent or weak cough reflex or are unable to cough effectively. It is particularly important that they are *not* fed with their head tipped back, as this facilitates the passage of food into the airway.

If particular foods or drinks are liable to induce gagging, choking or vomiting this should be investigated and alternatives should be provided. Young children, and older ones who have difficulty in eating or drinking, should never be given nuts or boiled sweets. Foods of this type and similar shapes and textures may lead to choking. Aspiration (breathing in food or drink) is a common problem which, when small amounts are involved, does not usually present a significant problem. However, persistent aspiration can lead to recurrent chest infections and should be fully investigated. It is important to check that the palate (roof of the mouth) is clear of food following a meal as residual food could lead to later choking if left in place.

People who feed children should be taught how to deal with a child who is choking. First aid courses are run by organizations such as the British Red Cross and St John Ambulance Brigade (*see Appendix IV*) as well as at local colleges. In-service training may be provided in schools, health centres and hospitals.

In general, if a baby or child chokes, bring his head, shoulders and body forward. If the obstruction is clearly visible, try to hook it out of the mouth using your finger. If the obstruction is not dislodged, a young baby may be held by his feet upside down and given a sharp slap between the shoulder blades. Should this not successfully dislodge the obstruction, repeat the procedure up to three more times. An older baby or child should be put face down over your lap or knees and given a sharp slap between the shoulder blades. Should this not successfully dislodge the obstruction, repeat the procedure up to three more times.

If this is not successful a technique called the abdominal thrust is recommended. Seek advice from appropriately trained people on its use.

If you are unsuccessful in clearing the obstruction get immediate assistance from a trained first-aider, nurse or doctor and call for an ambulance.

Please note that advice on giving first aid does change. The reader should seek expert advice on dealing with the child or baby who is choking to ensure that up-to-date information is utilized.

Cases of children who cough or choke persistently should be investigated by a doctor, as these signs indicate that swallowing is not co-ordinated. Techniques for observing and identifying eating/drinking and swallowing movements may be recommended. These include videofluoroscopy, radio-isotope and Barium swallows. These involve the baby or child being given food or liquid containing either radioactive or other material which can then be viewed under X-ray to provide information which is interpreted by a radiologist (a specialist in the interpretation of X-rays). It is important to discuss the use of such techniques with the team caring for the child. Whilst these investigations can be useful, they will not always be recommended by the child's doctor.

Because the protective cough reflex is so important, it may be useful for children who have a weak cough reflex to be seen by a physiotherapist. She may be able to demonstrate and teach other people to carry out chest-clearing procedures such as postural drainage, tapping and suctioning where necessary.

Safety procedures often recommended for staff feeding children include wearing protective gloves and being vaccinated against hepatitis 'B'. Staff should consult their managers regarding local policy on safety precautions.

Monitoring

This refers to the need to re-evaluate the child's eating and drinking skills constantly. Each snack or meal provides the opportunity to do this in an informal way. *Continuing assessment is part of therapy.*

Time

Do give both the child and feeder/assistant *time to adapt* to new ideas. One of the features of cerebral palsy is the difficulty in adapting from one pattern of movement to another. This applies to the more obvious shifts, such as moving from sitting to standing, as well as to patterns involving smaller movements, such as changing from sucking to chewing.

Feeding children may take a very long time, perhaps two hours or more. This is not usually helpful, for several reasons. Eating may be very tiring for the child both physically and emotionally. Prolonged mealtimes are equally hard for whoever is feeding the child. Lengthy meals make it unlikely that the child will be hungry when next offered food. Food often becomes less appetizing as it becomes cold and its texture may change. Children usually take most food during the first 40 minutes or so. It is therefore usually appropriate to reduce the time spent on a meal to perhaps an hour maximum. By assessing how much food is then taken, the feeder can judge if this will significantly reduce the child's intake.

If there is concern regarding adequate nutrition, the advice of a dietician should be sought. Supplements may be recommended so that the child is able to take in more calories without having to eat more food. See Chapter 8 for further information.

◆ PRACTICAL EXERCISE 12

This is to highlight the complex nature of mealtimes and the need to allow time for change.

Imagine you are four years old and have difficulty eating and drinking. You are about to stay at school for lunch for the first time. You have been used to being fed by your mother in your special chair in the kitchen at home. You live in a quiet road and your big sister is usually at school at lunchtime. Sometimes the television or cassette player is on and you have several rests during lunch to play. What is it like at school? The first obvious difference is the noise. You can hear a lot of adults and children talking. Someone is crying, someone else has dropped a plate on the floor. You are not in your usual chair. You are being fed by a stranger who is also feeding another child. She is feeding you far too quickly and you feel as if you are going to choke. She does not understand your attempts to communicate. How do you feel? You might feel overwhelmed by the sudden disruption to your life.

Such a child may well require help at mealtimes and changes will be required. However, *time must be given* to enable the child and feeder to feel comfortable with each other and the new surroundings. Any alterations to the feeding set-up should be approached in *very small steps*. Thorough, clear *explanations* should be given to ensure effective carry over. Regular check-ups, ideally at least once a week to start with, should occur to provide reassurance and encouragement and appropriate treatment. *Sensitivity, caring, trust and know-how* make up the basis for successful therapy. New ideas or seating are often best introduced *outside mealtimes*, when there is less pressure: after all, you would not practise running only when rushing to catch a train. Mid-morning or afternoon snacktimes are often suitable starting points. The child is usually not tired and there is *less pressure* on the child and whoever is feeding him to provide a specific intake of food or drink.

PRACTICAL MANAGEMENT

Sensation and perception

Sensation is the ability of our sensory organs, that is, eyes, skin, tongue, muscles, nose and ears, to receive information. The ears are involved with both hearing and balance. Proprioceptors in the muscles and joints enable us to know where each part of our body is and how it is moving. Perception is the ability of the brain to process and interpret the sensory message. Difficulties in these areas can seriously affect the eating and drinking process. These difficulties can be divided into several categories.

Hypersensitivity

This is where the child appears to have a *stronger reaction* to a specific sensation than would be expected. Hypersensitivity is related to lack of experience which is in turn related to lack of movement. For example, the child's inability to put his hands and toys to his mouth may have led to fearfulness of oral stimuli. This may be seen, for example, as exaggerated mouth opening on hearing the microwave beeps in anticipation of being fed. Other signs of hypersensitivity may include pushing into extension, tightening of lips, turning away, gagging or vomiting. Where a child has a history of being tube-fed he may react with grimacing and crying when food is reintroduced into the mouth. However, it should be remembered that we have all experienced hypersensitivity to certain stimuli, as when particular smells cause nausea or when we 'jump' on hearing an unexpected sound when we are already feeling tense.

Hyposensitivity

This is where the child appears to show *less reaction* to specific stimuli than expected. For example, the child may not be aware of where food is inside his mouth. The hypotonic (floppy) child may appear not to respond to stimuli, not because he has not seen, heard and so on but because his reactions are limited because of low muscle tone.

Careful assessment is required as it is possible for a child with hypersensitivity to 'block' or defend himself so much from sensation that he *appears* unresponsive. Sensitivity is often compounded by emotional factors such as fear and environmental factors such as a noisy room.

Note that a child with a visual impairment may not be ready to accept the spoon because *poor sight* has prevented anticipatory steps such as mouth opening from occurring.

Sensory defensiveness

For some children, the ability to discriminate the real nature of their sensory input is impaired. The tactile (touch) system both protects us and informs us. Protective reactions make us strike out or withdraw (fight or flight) but the informative aspect of the touch system helps us to explore and learn. In the child who is tactile defensive, the gentle touch of a soothing arm may be felt as pain or discomfort, so that the child pulls away, or seems 'stuck' in a protective 'mode' and cannot enjoy the sensation and learn from it.

Some children become defensive as a result of poor handling and environmental factors, particularly if they are totally blind.

The child may be particularly defensive to stimulation in and around the mouth (oral defensiveness), to sounds (auditory defensiveness) or movement.

Sensory overload

We learn to identify all the stimuli that bombard the body. We learn to attend to those that are relevant and filter out those that are unimportant at any one time; that is, we learn to sift and integrate sensory information. For example, while talking to a friend we do not notice an aeroplane passing overhead; however, we would not listen to our friend if we were plane spotting! While sleeping we do not wake to meaningless sounds such as traffic (for town dwellers) but wake instantly on hearing our baby.

Infants and children have to learn to filter stimuli in order to focus on important information. Where this sifting mechanism is faulty the child often exhibits distractibility and hyperactivity. Attention may flit during a meal; for example, a picture on the wall may distract the child from the food on the table. It is possible that a child will show more than one reaction, such as both hypersensitivity and sensory defensiveness.

Advice from a therapist with post-graduate training and experience in sensory integration should be sought where possible. (See *Appendix IV*.)

Normalizing sensation (sometimes known as 'desensitization')

This describes the process through which the child is helped to accept and tolerate stimuli that were previously rejected. The child becomes able to modulate his response appropriately. In the hyposensitive child, the aim is to increase sensory awareness — the term 'desensitization' is therefore inappropriate in such instances.

As the mouth is a very sensitive part of our body and as it is the focus of eating and drinking, it is not surprising that it is often in this place that the child finds it most difficult to tolerate touch. Neurologically, there is a close connection between the hands and mouth and many children with cerebral palsy are hypersensitive in these areas. They may not have been able to explore objects, food or utensils with their hands or mouth, so gradual and carefully selected steps in providing these experiences will be important. Therapists may be able to offer helpful advice.

It is essential that we do not inadvertently make the situation worse by inappropriate handling of the child. We should be aware of the child's reactions and be prepared and able to alter or even stop what we are doing if necessary. The following guidelines are suggested. However, it should be stressed that some children may not accept stimulation as easily as others. Be prepared to stop and seek advice, preferably from a therapist who has received recognized training in this field of work.

1 The child should be well positioned in a stable, comfortable way which ensures that the head is upright and in mid-line (symmetrical alignment) with an elongated back of neck as shown, for example, in Figure 10. The child's mouth should be closed if possible.

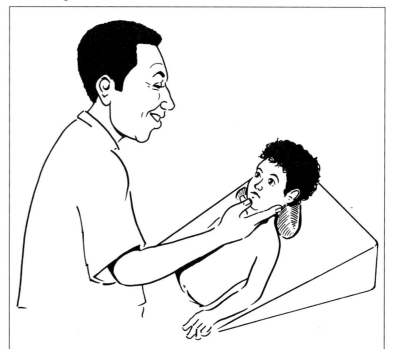

Figure 10 *An example of a good lying position*
Note: The child is well supported and calm; he is symmetrical; his neck is elongated; his arm is relaxed; the adult is providing oral control; there is good eye contact between them.

2 Start by touching the child on a part of the body where this is readily accepted and tolerated. This may be the child's arms, legs or body.

This is to enable you to differentiate the effects of light and firm touch.

Lightly stroke your hard palate (roof of the mouth) with the tip of your tongue. How does it feel? Now firmly rub your tongue against the palate. Which feels more pleasant or more uncomfortable? Most people find that light pressure feels tickly and uncomfortable, whereas firmer pressure is more acceptable.

3   In general when touching the child you should use firm, rhythmical, slow, stroking movements *towards the body*, if touching the limbs, or *towards the face*, if touching the body. Use your hands (warmed), a flannel or towelling. It is *very* important that the pressure is very firm or heavy, *without* causing pain or skin reddening.

4   Try to keep these movements symmetrical.

5   *Stop as soon as the child shows any sign of distress*, such as pushing back, blinking or retracting (pulling up) the upper lip.

6   Treat it as a relaxed playing time for fun, not an exercise.

7   Do it for short periods of time, up to several times a day if possible. Even as little as one minute is very effective. Only do it before meals or snacks when the child clearly enjoys it.

8   Playing soothing music or singing gently may help.

9   It is usually easier for the child to tolerate his own fingers in his mouth. Help him to do this, but be careful to prevent him biting his fingers. (This activity may not be recommended for children who habitually put their hands to their mouth.) The child can also put his fingers in his parents' mouths. A physiotherapist or occupational therapist will be able to suggest how such movements may be accomplished.

10 When touching the face, aim to move *symmetrically towards the mouth* to encourage lip closure. (See Figure 11.) Go slowly: some children strongly dislike this. Remember that some children are unable to breathe through the nose because of

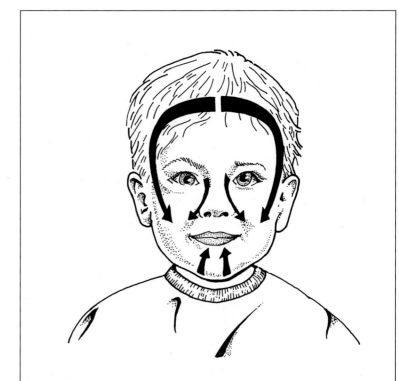

Figure 11 *Move the hands symmetrically towards the mouth*
Note: When touching the face, move your hands symmetrically towards the mouth, as shown by the arrows.

nasal blockage and so on. Do watch for signs of distress and release lip closure if necessary.

11 Before touching around or inside the mouth, remember to wash your hands. (As a precaution, many health and education authorities either recommend or insist that staff wear gloves — similar to those worn by dentists — before any such activity.)

12 Stimulation inside the mouth needs to be carried out with particular care. Fingernails should be kept short. For under-fives, the adult's little finger is the most appropriate size. For most older children the adult's index finger is better, although the relative size of the adult's hand and the child's mouth should be considered.

13 Always wet the finger before using it, as this is more
comfortable. Place the padded part *just off centre* towards the
side best tolerated by the child, then roll it inside the upper lip
and firmly massage the upper gums to the side, then go back
to the starting point. (See Figures 12a, 12b and 12c). Do not
go too far back at first or the child may gag. Repeat up to three
times if the child accepts this. Do this at a speed that is best
tolerated by the child. Repeat to the other side of the upper
gums, then the opposite side's lower gums, then the remaining
side's lower gums. Keep the mouth as closed as possible
during this activity (see Oral control, pages 56–7).

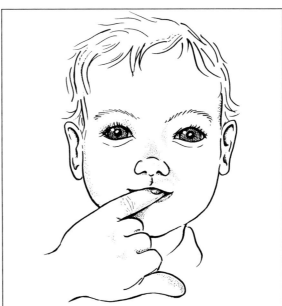

Figure 12b *Introduce your finger into the child's mouth 2*
Note: Roll your finger inside the lip, so that your fingernail now
touches it.

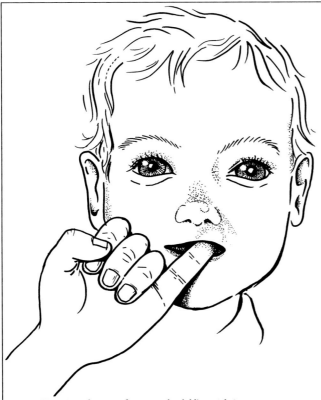

Figure 12a *Introduce your finger into the child's mouth 1*
Note: Place the pad of your little finger inside the lip — your fingernail
is towards the child's gum/teeth.

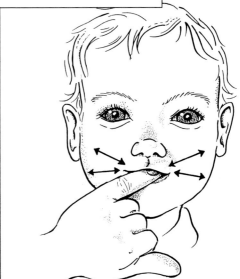

Figure 12c *Gum massage*
Note: Massage the gums systematically, one-quarter of the mouth
at a time.

The Practical Management of Eating & Drinking Difficulties in Children

14 You can massage inside the cheeks by pulling them out gently, then massaging in a circular motion. (See Figure 13.) Both massaging activities increase saliva production and it is important that you give the child the opportunity to swallow as necessary. Oral (jaw) control, as described later, is often helpful. This helps to develop saliva control, thus reducing dribbling as well as increasing tolerance to oral stimulation.

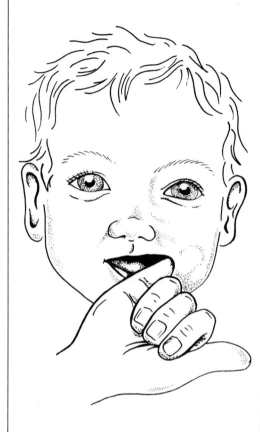

Figure 13 *Cheek massage*
Note: Massage inside the cheeks, using your finger in a circular motion.

15 Enabling the child to mouth toys such as teething toys, his and your own fingers and so on provides helpful experiences.

16 If the child's teeth are not being cleaned, this should be investigated. 'Therapeutic' toothbrushing is described in Chapter 9 and is strongly recommended. The same chapter gives ideas regarding appropriate oral hygiene if a child will not tolerate a toothbrush.

17 Once the child will tolerate oral touch more easily you can introduce extra stimuli by slightly wetting your finger with liquids such as fruit juice or milk. The child may need time to adapt to this increased stimulation. Do not continue if the child shows distress or has difficulty in coping with this additional stimulation, for example if he splutters, coughs or cries.

18 Water play with cups and spoons may be helpful. Bath times may be suitable for such games. Bowls of water will also provide useful opportunities for fun and learning. Be cautious and aware that some babies and children will not be able to cope with splashes or larger quantities of liquid that enter the mouth in play.

19 'Pretend' play involving dolls and teddies having tea parties may be helpful for some children.

20 Playing with food, such as finger painting with tomato ketchup or yogurt can be helpful but should not be continued if the child dislikes it. Physiotherapists and occupational therapists may be able to advise further on this area.

Jaw and mouth stability (oral control)

As described earlier, the normal development of eating and drinking is dependent on the child's physical development. Head control and the ability to keep the jaw reasonably stable are prerequisites for mature chewing and drinking. Many children with cerebral palsy have great difficulty in maintaining an upright head and trunk position. The mouth may be constantly open or there may be difficulty in grading jaw movement, so that any attempt to open the mouth results in a wide open position, or 'too much' opening.

Where this lack of jaw stability or poor grading of jaw movement occurs, it is often very helpful for the feeder to provide this stability using her arm and hand. This approach is referred to as oral or jaw control. It is important that *the child is in a good position*; that is, the

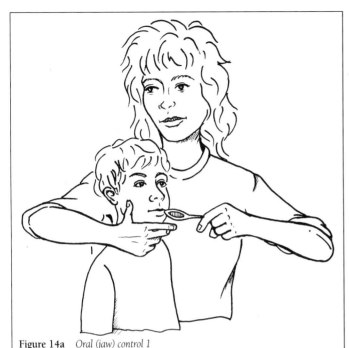

Figure 14a *Oral (jaw) control 1*
Note: The child's head is upright, supported by the adult's shoulder.

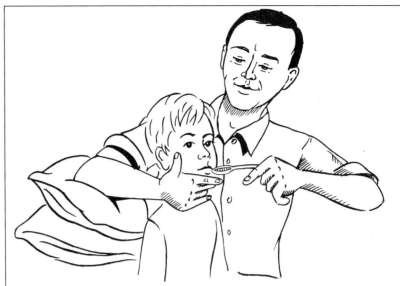

Figure 14c *Oral (jaw) control 3*
Note: The child's head is upright, supported by the adult's shoulder; the adult rests his elbow on cushions as he has long arms.

head and trunk should be in alignment *before* oral control is used. The feeder should provide *firm* control, but it should feel comfortable. The feeder's arm is placed behind the child's neck so that the upper part or crook of her arm, or her shoulder, may be used to elongate the back of the child's neck. (See Figures 14a and 14b).

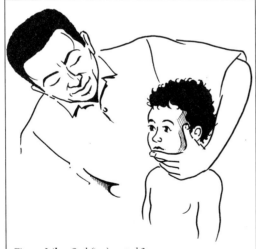

Figure 14b *Oral (jaw) control 2*
Note: The child's head is upright; the adult is using oral control.

If the feeder has long arms, she may be more comfortable if she rests her elbow on a pillow placed on an adjacent table and fills the space between her arm and the child's head and neck with a rolled up towel or something similar, making sure that elongation of the back of the neck is maintained. (See Figure 14c.)

To begin with, oral control should be used *between meals*, to accustom the child to it. The child could be sitting, lying down or standing as long as the principles of head and trunk alignment with an elongated back of neck are observed. (See Figures 6a–c, and 10.) It can be used with babies as well, although, as with the child, it should not be continued if the baby shows distress or discomfort. If the baby or child has a blocked up nose, *do not* keep the mouth closed, as breathing may be difficult. Keep the child happy while using oral control by singing, reading a story, watching television together and so on. However, avoid overstimulating the child as this may make it more difficult for him to remain calm.

The Practical Management of Eating & Drinking Difficulties in Children

Feeding from the side

The child needs to be in a stable position with an upright head and trunk position. Always sit so that you encourage maximum normal activity of the most affected side. The physiotherapist or occupational therapist can advise. (See Figures 15a, 15b and 15c).

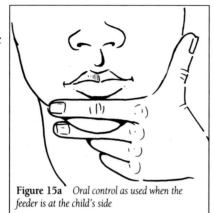

Figure 15a   *Oral control as used when the feeder is at the child's side*

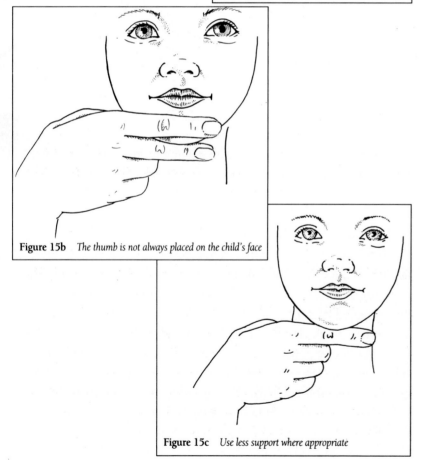

Figure 15b   *The thumb is not always placed on the child's face*

Figure 15c   *Use less support where appropriate*

Feeder's middle finger

Use this finger with the padded part up. It should be placed under the mouth just behind the bony part of the chin. This encourages the child's tongue to come down and stay down, enabling the child to swallow in a more mature way. It also assists mouth closure and reduces tongue protrusion.

Feeder's index finger

Place the padded part of this finger on the chin below the lower lip. Avoid touching the lip as this prevents the child from using it actively. *Do not rest the other fingers on the child's throat*, as this restricts movement and may cause gagging. Using the finger in this way helps to elongate the back of the neck and to keep the chin slightly tucked in. It helps to stabilize the lower lip and may also assist in mouth opening.

Feeder's thumb

Rest the thumb on the child's cheek near the ear, or hold it slightly away from that part of the face if it is not needed to help the child or stabilize the feeder's hand. Do not leave it near the child's eye as this may distract or irritate him. It may also help to prevent jaw deviation: for example, if the child's jaw tends to move to the right, the presence of the feeder's thumb on the right cheek may inhibit that pattern.

The fingers should be kept straight to prevent the tips from pushing into the child's face. Care should be taken to prevent the feeder pulling the child towards her, or tipping the child's head back during feeding.

Feeding from the front

The child needs to be in a stable position with an elongated back of neck. This may be achieved using items such as a rolled towel or neck cushion.

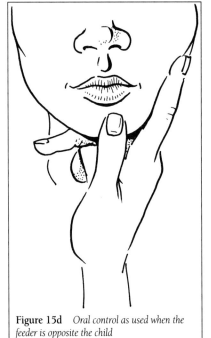

Figure 15d *Oral control as used when the feeder is opposite the child*

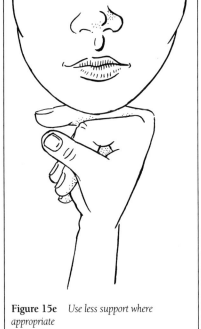

Figure 15e *Use less support where appropriate*

Feeder's middle finger

Place a middle finger under the jaw just behind the chin. (See Figures 15d and 15e). This will assist mouth closure, reduce tongue protrusion and keep the tongue down rather than pushed against the roof of the mouth.

Feeder's index finger

The index finger should be held straight along the line of the jaw to the ear. The pad of the fingertip rests in front of the earlobe. Do not use it if it is not necessary. This will stabilize the feeder's hand.

Feeder's thumb

Place the thumb on the chin below the lower lip; avoid touching the lower lip, as this prevents the child from using it actively. You will find that this helps to elongate the back of the child's neck and to keep the chin slightly tucked in. It also assists mouth opening and helps to stabilize the lower lip.

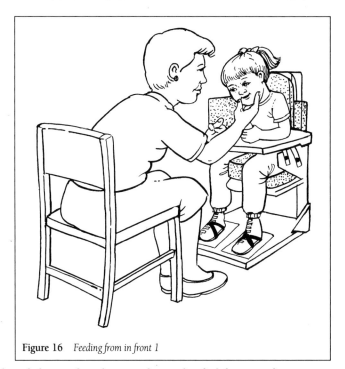

Figure 16 *Feeding from in front 1*

The child with better head control may be fed from in front. (See Figure 16.) When feeding from the front, care should be taken not to tip the child's head backward, especially when food is placed into the mouth.

Remember: The child may not require such help throughout the whole meal. It may only be needed for a short time. Pressure may be released as the child develops more control. For example, help may be required specifically for drinking or for eating soft foods, or it may only be needed to assist mouth opening. Support with one finger or thumb may be all that is required. This approach can take a while to get used to: the feeder and child require time to adjust and initially it should be tried *outside mealtimes*. Extra care is required if the feeder has long fingernails. (They may need to be cut.) It is a good idea to practise this on other adults and children who do not have physical disabilities. You can then tell each other how it felt so that you are confident in its use before using it with children who require such

The Practical Management of Eating & Drinking Difficulties in Children

support. If it is possible for someone to help you, ask her to photograph or video you when you are doing it well. This provides a very useful reminder for anyone feeding that child.

Bite reflex

There are two types of bite reflex, the normal phasic bite reflex and the abnormal bite reflex. They are sometimes confused but can be differentiated as follows:

	BITE REFLEX	NORMAL PHASIC BITE REFLEX
Type of reflex	An abnormal reflex. It is probably a spasm of the masseter (jaw) muscle	A normal reflex gradually replaced by a volitional bite at 3–5 months
Muscle tone	Increased	Normal
Effect of position	Associated with flexion (bending forward), ie more likely if the child is bent forwards with arms flexed and hands fisted. More likely to be stimulated if spoon and so on presented centrally	Not associated with specific position
Initiated	Usually starts suddenly and bite *becomes stronger*	Starts suddenly but *released quickly*
Jaw movement	Clenched hard	Firm closure followed by prompt opening
Occurrence	Both may occur in response to food entering the mouth. A bite reflex may be associated with hypersensitivity. When a child typically responds to food or drink by using a bite reflex this prevents more independent movement of the jaw, lips and tongue.	

Management

As a bite reflex is part of a pattern of flexion, the first step may be to put the child in a more extended position. The child's hips should be *slightly* extended and the head or trunk should be *slightly* rotated, that is turned to one side. This helps to break up the symmetry and thus inhibit the onset of a bite reflex. Ask a physiotherapist, occupational therapist or speech and language therapist for advice if necessary. Food should be presented *slightly* to one side of the mouth, for the same reason.

Develop chewing skills. Where possible offer finger-fed food to the sides of the mouth, as described on page 63. This is preferable to spoon-feeding as the child may bite on the spoon. Therapeutic toothbrushing is helpful (*see Chapter 9 for details*). Normalize sensation (see page 53 for details).

If a child uses a bite reflex, the following may be tried:

1 Wait for the spasm to pass spontaneously.
2 Push up under the chin, using your finger.
3 Firmly tap one side of the jaw.
4 *Slightly* rotate and extend the child's body — ask a physiotherapist or occupational therapist for advice.

The following are usually counter-productive and are *not* recommended: attempting to prise the jaw open or trying to pull anything out of the mouth that is caught between the teeth, both of which may make the child bite down even harder. Showing emotions such as anxiety and anger may increase the child's muscle tone and perpetuate the spasm.

Tongue thrust

This is sometimes confused with sucking. The two can be differentiated as follows:

	TONGUE THRUST	SUCKING
Type of reflex	Abnormal	Normal — the forward/backward tongue movement is replaced by a more mature up/down pattern by approximately nine–twelve months
Muscle tone	Increased	Normal
Appearance of tongue	Thick and bunched	Flattish with rounded end
Effect of position	Associated with extension, ie more likely if child pushes back with head back. More likely to be stimulated if spoon or food is presented centrally	Not associated with specific position
Rhythm	Not rhythmical	Rhythmical
Initiated	Often starts suddenly	Begins easily and smoothly
Tongue protrusion	May protrude far beyond mouth	Usually protrudes no further than just beyond the lips
Jaw movement	Often *very* wide	Opens, but not excessively

Both tongue thrust and sucking may occur in anticipation of food but may also be seen outside mealtimes, either involuntarily or as a way of indicating hunger or thirst. A child may exhibit both patterns. When a child's typical oral movement pattern is sucking and/or tongue thrusting this *overactivity* of the tongue actually inhibits the development of more refined lip and tongue activity.

Management

As tongue thrusting is so often part of a pattern of extension the first step is to handle and position the child so as to inhibit extension or extensor spasms. This involves hip flexion (bending slightly forward) bringing the shoulders forward, bending the knees and keeping the feet flat on the floor or foot-rest. The arms should be brought forward, ideally resting on the table (where one is used).

The back of the neck should be elongated and the head supported in mid-line (symmetrical alignment), using oral control, as described earlier. (See Figure 5.) The feeder should not be too high up; nor should food be presented from high up, or the child's gaze towards her/it could lead to extension.

Use oral (jaw) control as described to prevent the jaw from opening too soon or too wide. Move the middle finger up and slightly back against the forward movement of the tongue which usually accompanies jaw opening.

The use of spoon pressure can help to inhibit tongue thrusting. This is described on page 65. Avoid giving runny or soft food by spoon, as this increases tongue thrusting and sucking. Develop chewing skills (see next section for details). Stop or at least decrease the use of straws, dummies and bottles where possible as they reinforce sucking and tongue thrusting. Therapeutic toothbrushing is helpful (*see Chapter 9 for details*).

Developing chewing skills

As explained in Chapter 2, chewing normally starts to develop from six to nine months. Remember that biting is an integral part of chewing and that vertical 'munching' precedes chewing. It is therefore essential to work on a child's biting skills in order to develop chewing. Lateral tongue movements are required for chewing. As more skill is required to eat food combinations, chewing practice should be introduced using a single-textured food.

Position

It is very important to ensure that the child is well positioned. In order for the more complex oral skills required for chewing to develop, a mid-line (symmetrical alignment) upright head and trunk, elongated back of neck and slightly tucked-in chin are essential (see Figure 5). Oral control may be required to provide head and mouth stability (see pages 56–60 for details). Initially the practice sessions should be restricted to non-mealtime situations, so that there is *no* pressure on the child to eat what is presented or on the feeder to make the child eat.

New foods should be introduced in small amounts. For example, when offered as part of a meal, just a little of the new food can be presented next to the more familiar foods. 'Pretend' eating using a doll's or teddy's tea party may be helpful with children of an appropriate age or developmental level; however, it is not appropriate for young children with a visual impairment.

Stages in improving chewing skills

The following information provides some guidelines for developing chewing skills. There will be overlap and the child is not expected to progress strictly from one stage to the next. When introducing new foods to meals, it is usually best to do so at whichever meal is the most successful.

Stage 1 aims to stimulate biting or munching and lateral tongue movements. It is usually best to start with rubber teething toys with suitably shaped protuberances or foods that will not break up, such as a stick of liquorice, a dried peach, or a strip of cooked beef (*see Appendix II*). Where the child is too old to make the use of such toys acceptable, or where the feeder is unsure whether or not the child might be able to bite off a piece of food that is then a potential danger, it is advisable to use the 'muslin pouch' technique.

Take a clean, small, thin cotton handkerchief or similar-sized piece of muslin. *Do not* use gauze, as the threads sometimes come loose. Place a small piece of food in the centre of the muslin and continue as shown in Figure 17. In general select softer foods, such as banana or ripe peeled pear, for a child with a stiff mouth and firmer food, such as dried apricot or liquorice, for a child with athetosis or a floppy mouth. Alter the size of the piece of food according to the size of the child's mouth. Too large a piece may cause gagging and too small a piece may not provide enough sensory information to which the child is able to respond. Twist the material around the food to form a pouch which should be moistened, using water or another acceptable liquid. This will make it feel more pleasant to the child. The feeder holds the 'handle' and keeps hold of it to prevent the child from taking in too much. Whether using a

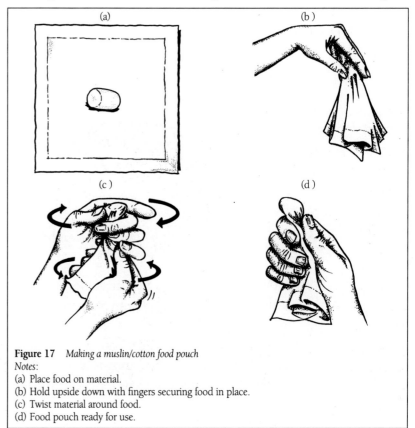

Figure 17 *Making a muslin/cotton food pouch*
Notes:
(a) Place food on material.
(b) Hold upside down with fingers securing food in place.
(c) Twist material around food.
(d) Food pouch ready for use.

The Practical Management of Eating & Drinking Difficulties in Children

toy, a piece of firm food or the pouch, proceed as follows.

Providing oral control as necessary, start by placing the item to *whichever* side of the child's mouth moves *more normally*. This is usually the same side as the more able side of the body. Make sure that the item is placed along the line of the jaw, as shown in Figure 18a. Placement as in Figure 18b causes the lips to be pulled apart. Placement as in Figure 18c crosses the mid-line and may stimulate sucking, tongue thrusting or biting. Do not go too far back, as you may cause gagging (retching). Children who do not chew often have a very sensitive gag reflex, so great care must be taken. Abnormal muscle tone can

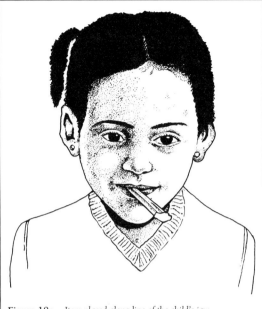

Figure 18a   *Item placed along line of the child's jaw*

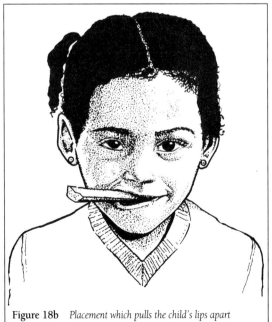

Figure 18b   *Placement which pulls the child's lips apart*

make it difficult for the child to gag. It is therefore important to watch the child for *signs of gagging*, such as glazed or watering eyes, blinking or eye closing. Do give the child *time* to respond, then place the item to the *other* side of the child's mouth to provide bilateral stimulation. If the child bites down, but does not show any further activity, try

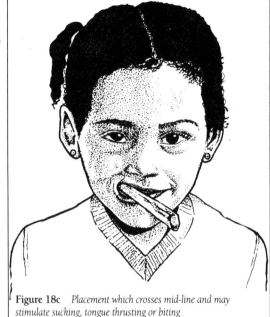

Figure 18c   *Placement which crosses mid-line and may stimulate sucking, tongue thrusting or biting*

pulling the item *gently*, or pressing the food down then waiting, to provide resistance which may stimulate a biting movement. Check that the child does not bite a hole in the pouch.

When using toys, or a firm piece of food, it may be helpful to try dipping the item into fruit juice, or smooth foods such as yogurt or fruit purée before presenting it to the child. This will obviously provide more stimulation and greater salivation, *so more oral control may be required*. Once the child is able to bite more easily, go on to the second stage.

Stage 2 aims to stimulate biting off a piece of food and using lateral tongue movements. Strips of food which are easy to bite and dissolve easily should be presented to alternate sides, as described above. Suitable foods include prawn crackers, 'Wotsits' (or similar), 'Quavers' (or similar), sponge finger biscuits and cream-filled wafer biscuits (*see Appendix II*). Make sure that the child is *not given too much at once*. Again, *time* should be given to enable the child to respond. If the child is unable to bite off the food, the feeder can

The Practical Management of Eating & Drinking Difficulties in Children

assist by breaking it off. Once the child is able to bite off such foods a variety of them can be offered as regular snacks at the beginning of meals, and the next stage may be introduced.

Stage 3 aims to stimulate munching and lateral tongue movement in early chewing. Strips of food that are easy to bite and chew should be presented to alternate sides, as described above. Care should again be taken to place the food along the jaw line and not so far back as to cause gagging (see earlier). Suitable foods include the following: peeled fresh ripe pear (or tinned), soft boiled root vegetables and pasta (without sauce) (*see Appendix II*). These foods can be given as snacks and can form part of the child's meals where possible. These textures should replace soft, spoon-fed foods where possible, so that the child has more opportunities to practise chewing and less to reinforce sucking.

It takes time, thought and imagination to look at meal presentation in a different way. Some examples of possible changes are:

USUAL	NEW IDEA
Mashed potato	Strips of well cooked boiled potato
Fruit purée	Strips of peeled ripe pear
Sponge cake and custard	Cake given dry in 'fingers'. Custard can be diluted and drunk. (See *Developing Drinking Skills*, pages 65–69.)

You will have noticed that finger-feeding, that is the feeder presenting food using her fingers, is described in preference to spoon-feeding. This is because it stimulates biting and chewing, whereas spoon-feeding may reinforce sucking, tongue thrusting or a bite reflex. The final stage can be introduced gradually.

Stage 4 aims to provide further opportunity for chewing. Foods which are moderately easy to chew can be introduced. These include cheese, well cooked fish and poultry (*see Appendix II*).

Improving spoon-feeding
General points

1   If the child is only sucking and not chewing, it is *important to give food of an even texture*. If lumps are mixed with gravy, for example, the child may swallow pieces whole (which is not good for digestion) or *may choke*. He may spit out the lumps, which reinforces sucking and tongue thrusting, as described earlier.

2   *Keep food dry*. Once it combines with saliva it will form a suitable consistency. If food is moist to start with it quickly becomes runny once inside the mouth, which often increases sucking and leads to greater food loss. Piling it high on the end of the spoon makes food removal easier for the child.

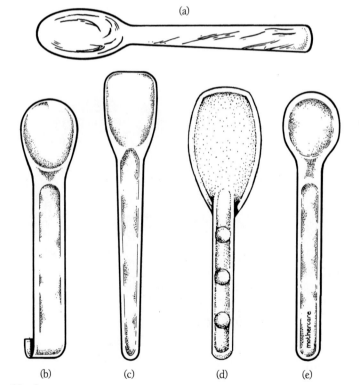

Figure 19 *Spoons*
Note: (a) Bone; (b) Boots; (c) Cheyne spoon (small); (d) Cheyne spoon (large); (e) Mothercare.

3 *Use a small, shallow spoon with a rounded or 'shovel-shaped' bowl.* (It is harder to remove food from a deep spoon — try it yourself.) *Strong, plastic* material is usually the most comfortable if the child has a bite reflex (as described earlier); such spoons are available, for example, at Mothercare and Boots; and the *Cheyne* polythene spoons are also useful (see *Appendix I* and Figure 19). A similarly shaped metal spoon, such as a mustard or ice cream spoon, may be acceptable.

If the spoon is too large for the child's mouth it will touch the teeth and may be uncomfortable. It is important to select the spoon carefully (*see Chapter 6*). Ask an occupational therapist, physiotherapist or speech and language therapist for advice, especially when independent eating is being established.

4 Bring the spoon slowly to the child's mouth level, approaching from the front and slightly below the child's eye level. Bringing the spoon from above may lead the child to look up and go into extension (push back). Use oral control to grade mouth opening. (Do not allow the mouth to open wide, as this may lead to extension in the neck and body.) Press the spoon onto the front of the tongue. This helps to prevent tongue thrusting. Keep it flat or the tip may push into the child's tongue. Tilt the child's head forward a little and allow time for the upper lip to move down before assisting mouth closure, using your hand where necessary. Withdraw the spoon between the lips. Do this slowly to give the child time to adapt. If the child does not use his upper lip, try raising the spoon to enable him to feel the food on the lip, then proceed as above.

5 If the food is soft, once it is in the mouth, tongue movements and swallowing can be facilitated using

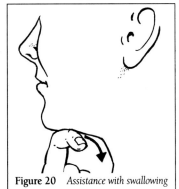

Figure 20 *Assistance with swallowing*

the feeder's middle finger beneath the jaw. Move it slowly and rhythmically up and back between the point of the chin and the angle of the neck where the floor of the mouth joins the neck. (See Figure 20.)

Try not to scrape food from the spoon against the child's top teeth or gums. There are several reasons for avoiding this: it prevents the child from using the top lip actively; it may make the child go into extension; it reinforces sucking or tongue thrusting and food tends to become lodged in the palate (roof of the mouth). Whether feeding by hand or by spoon, remember to consider and vary the following as appropriate:

◆ rate at which the child is fed,
◆ quantity that is offered,
◆ taste,
◆ temperature,
◆ texture.

Developing drinking skills

Liquid moves more quickly than solid food and it is often more difficult for children with cerebral palsy to drink than to eat. Adequate fluid intake is a major factor in the management of constipation and its importance cannot be overemphasized. Drinks should be offered regularly, usually more often than food. This is particularly important during hot weather.

As with the introduction of anything new, drinking practice should initially take place when there is no pressure to take fluid. Choose a time of day when the child and feeder are as relaxed as possible. Go slowly to give both partners time to adjust to the new ideas. Start with tastes and temperatures the baby or child likes the most.

Position of baby or child

As described in Chapter 5, the child's position is *fundamental* to the quality of his eating and drinking skills. Advice on positioning should be sought from the therapy team. In general the baby or child should be in an upright position with his head in alignment with his body. His head should be in mid-line (symmetrical alignment) with an elongated back of neck and a slightly tucked-in chin. (See Figures 21a and 21b.)

Breast-feeding

Where a mother wishes to breast-feed, it is probably most appropriate for her to discuss this with a breast feeding nurse or counsellor. Should the baby be unable to be breast-fed, the mother may wish to express milk to be taken by bottle or cup. This is beneficial to the baby and can be of psychological benefit to the mother, as she is thus able to contribute something very special to the care of her baby.

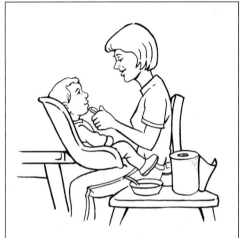

Figure 21a   *Feeding from in front 2*
Note: The baby is well supported in a seat; he is sitting symmetrically with his head in an upright position; there is body and face contact between adult and child; utensils and kitchen paper are close at hand

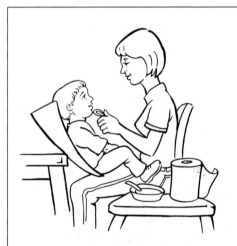

Figure 21b   *Feeding from in front 3*
Note: The baby is well supported on a wedge which is securely placed against a table which will remain stationary even if the child moves forcefully; there is body and face contact between adult and child; utensils and kitchen paper are close to hand

Bottle-feeding

In Chapter 6 we looked at several different types of bottles and teats. The appropriate one for a particular child will depend on the size and shape of the child's mouth and how easily and quickly he can drink. Too large or long a teat may cause gagging (retching). An enlarged hole, or the presence of several holes, may lead to too fast a rate of flow, so that the baby or child is unable to cope. This often leads to coughing, spluttering and liquid loss. The bottle should also be comfortable for the feeder to hold.

If it is necessary to enlarge a hole, this should be done by cutting a cross over the hole rather than gouging out an enlarged hole. (See Figure 22.) This is because the 'cross cut' closes after sucking, thus preventing excessive liquid loss. It is widely recommended that *solids* are *not* put into bottles. Should feeds require thickening, there are alternatives available (*see Chapter 8 on nutrition*). Whilst sucking is a normal stage in feeding development, it is by no means essential that a child goes through this experience. However, it is important for the child to have the opportunity to explore different things with his mouth.

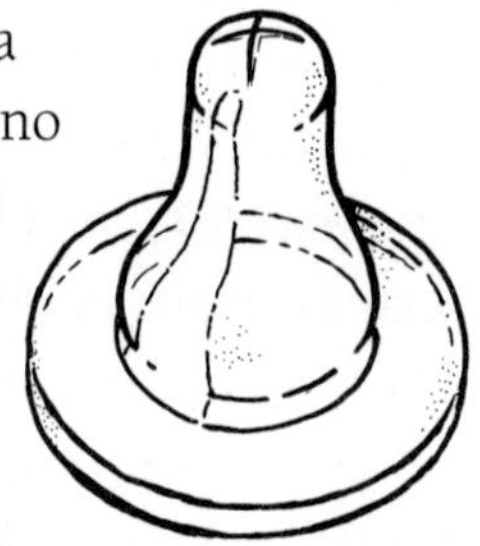

Figure 22   *A cross-cut teat*

If the baby is sucking in an abnormal way, trying to improve his bottle drinking if he is more than about four months old might not be advisable. Alternatively, try to wean him onto a small cup (see below). This is to enable him to learn something which will lead on to improved, more mature patterns. Once a baby can take a bottle well it is often extremely difficult to get him onto a cup. In the long term, extra time spent on developing cup drinking is usually well worth the effort.

Moving from bottle or breast to cup drinking

With regard to selecting a cup, see Chapter 6. A small, soft, flexible cup is best. Possibilities include:

◆ medicine holders, as used in hospitals (as long as the rim is not sharp);

◆ cups or jugs from children's teasets. Do ensure that they are made of a suitable, safe material;

◆ lids to feeding bottles;

◆ food storage containers.

Spouted cups may not be helpful, as they often lead to biting, or increased sucking or tongue thrusting. However, they do reduce spillage and their use should be fully discussed with appropriate members of the child's team. Where appropriate, a beaker such as the *Mothercare Variflow*, which enables the feeder to alter the rate of flow, may be helpful.

As described earlier, the baby or child should be *well positioned*, whether on the feeder's lap or on a chair. A physiotherapist, occupational therapist or speech and language therapist can advise on specific requirements depending on the child's age, physical needs and so on. In general the head should be upright with a lengthened back of neck. The head *should not be tipped back*. Stability may be given using an open

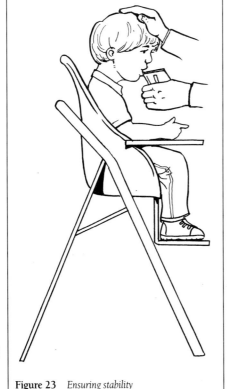

Figure 23   *Ensuring stability*

palm down onto the child's head; however *do not* tip back the child's head. (See Figure 23.)

Initially an empty cup can be introduced. A nice smelling drop of liquid or something like honey can be placed at the bottom and/or on the rim of the cup to get the child used to the smell and taste. Once this is accepted, offer a cup containing *smooth, thickened liquid* such as liquidized fruit purée (*see Appendix II*). Thick liquid moves more slowly than runny liquid, thus providing more sensory feedback, which makes it easier to control. Provide oral control as necessary to maintain lip closure until the cup rim is against the child's lips. With the rim gently resting on the lower lip, tip the cup so that the liquid moves slowly towards the mouth.

Do ensure that there is a lot of liquid present, or the child will have to wait too long for a drink and may become agitated. Be careful not to tip back the child's head as you tip a little liquid into the mouth. Give the child time to respond, using upper lip movement and sucking. It is important not to allow the tongue to thrust out between the lips and cup. Continue providing oral control during sucking if necessary, but do release your fingers if the child can cope more independently.

Extra help may be required to facilitate lip closure as the cup is removed. Initially the baby or child may only take a very small amount at a time. Once a child starts sucking, he may continue to do so in a reflex way. Whilst this is encouraging, the child may not be able to co-ordinate suck–swallow–breathe, so that sucking continues too long, leading to disorganized breathing. When the child is sucking, do ensure that you remove the cup every three sucks (or sooner) or so to enable the child to breathe. You might count aloud, "One, two, three, rest", to provide the idea of rhythm. *This timing is very important as breathing in while eating or drinking can lead to aspiration (inhalation of food or liquid) which can be very dangerous.*

This approach is also suitable for older children going on to a larger cup. When selecting a cup for an older child, the following points should be considered.

1 A flared rim can be helpful as it provides an anchor for the lower lip. (See Figure 24.)

2 A slanted cup such as a *Doidy* enables the feeder to see what the child is doing (see Figure 9a). It also prevents the child from feeling 'covered' by the cup, enables the child to see the feeder and is less likely to lead to the child's head being tipped back as he drinks.

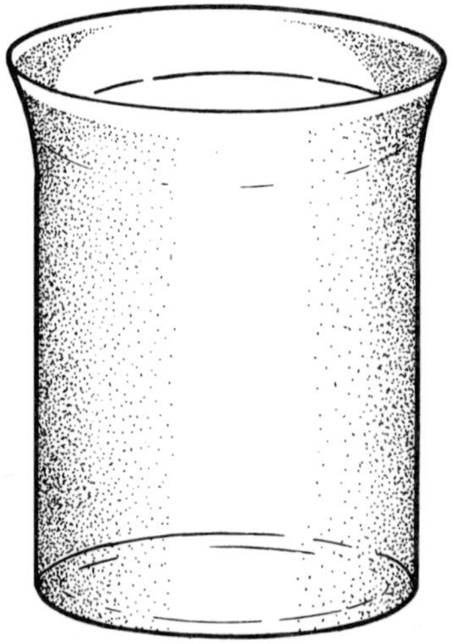

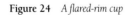

Figure 24   *A flared-rim cup*

3 A transparent cup such as the *Púr* has similar benefits to the *Doidy*. (See Figure 9b.)

4 A cup with a sunken lid and two medium holes or slits, such as the *Púr*, *Cheyne* and *MagMag*, provides a *central* point from which thick liquid can flow in a more controlled way (see Figures 9b, 9c and 9d) making it easier for the child to drink.

5 Where a spouted cup is used, holes can be enlarged, or melted and blocked, as required.

6 *The cup should not shatter or break if bitten.*

7 Considerations regarding independent drinking should be discussed with the therapists.

Straws

It is not usually appropriate to introduce straw drinking to a child who is not yet able to chew, particularly if the child has a tongue thrust. This is because the straw encourages a sucking pattern. Remember that children normally learn to use a straw several months after they have learnt to drink from a cup and chew. However, for some children it may be their only method of independent drinking.

Select the straws being used very carefully. A small gauge hole with thick walls will be easiest for children who are unable to suck well. Sometimes it is helpful to begin with wide, thick, plastic tubing (such as winemaking tubing) since (a) it is easier to form a seal around if lip rounding is a problem; (b) it does not collapse so easily; and (c) its translucency allows the feeder and child to see the level of the liquid.

Select a short length of tube (say 12 cm). Partially fill with liquid. Place your thumb over one end and place the tube between the child's lips. Remove your thumb briefly to release some liquid, thus stimulating oral movement. Where the child cannot cope with narrow tubing, build up the straws using wide tubing. Ask your occupational therapist for help. Putting something tasty around the top of the straw may help to encourage lip seal.

Packet fruit juices with inbuilt straws may be useful for children who are able to cope with such narrow straws. Otherwise, the straw could be replaced by a wider type. Straws can be similarly placed into a squeezable ketchup bottle. The adult can then exert pressure on the carton or bottle to assist the child.

The *MagMag* cup has a straw attachment. (*See Appendix I.*)

For children who have a very weak suck, the *Pat Saunders* straw, which has a valve to prevent the liquid falling back down when sucking stops, is very useful, but it is very narrow (see Figure 25). When sucking becomes established, various straws can be introduced such as narrower and longer varieties.

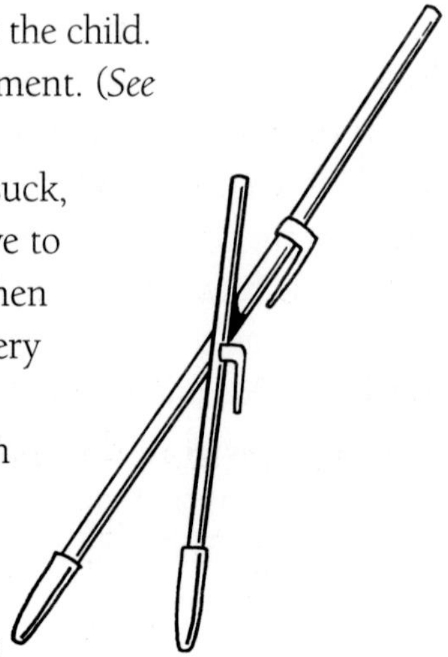

Figure 25   *Pat Saunders valved straws*

The Practical Management of Eating & Drinking Difficulties in Children

Whichever method of giving drinks is used, remember, as with food, to consider and vary the following as appropriate:

◆ rate at which drinks are given to the child,
◆ quantity which is given to the child,
◆ taste,
◆ temperature,
◆ consistency.

Sensory aspects

Many children with cerebral palsy have missed out on the normal stages of exploring objects with their hands and mouth. It is therefore important to provide the opportunity for finger play with foodstuffs in a safe, supervised manner such as finger painting with ketchup or yogurt and playing with dried pasta or large pieces of unsliced bread. *Do not let the child put anything in his mouth that could be dangerous.* This sort of play can be very messy. One parent sat her child in the bath (without water) and put a little ketchup around him. Once he had smeared it around and even tasted it, his mother showered him down!

It may be helpful to give children feeding utensils and cups that have only a small amount of food, such as honey, on them. A link between these items, *food smells* and possibly tastes can therefore be established in a play situation. Do not underestimate the effect of smells. They can provoke strong reactions of pleasure such as smiling and sucking. However, they can also induce unpleasant feelings such as nausea and *should be used with caution*.

The issue of self-feeding

How self-feeding normally develops

Babies and young children acquire the skills involved in self-feeding gradually over a period of several years (*see Chapter 2*). Early experience of putting hands to mouth, hands together, grasping an object and bringing it to the mouth takes place during the first three to four months. As the child acquires better head and trunk control, and in particular shoulder stability, he becomes more able to put his hands on a cup or bottle while he is being given a drink. He learns to finger-feed, hold a cup and then put a spoon to his mouth between nine and fourteen months. These skills require eye–hand co-ordination. The child then learns to load the spoon with food, to use a fork and, later still, a knife. With time and practice the child learns to grade (judge) movement more accurately. The child will normally play with his food and drink and will sometimes get himself as well as his immediate surroundings messy. Touching and exploring food and drink in this way is an important aspect of feeding development. Socially acceptable 'table manners' are taught as the child matures and will vary among different cultural groups. The baby or child takes several years to acquire these complex, highly co-ordinated skills. Remember that self-feeding is not normally established until the child is able to sit and chew well.

Self-feeding involves more than physical skills. The child has to be able to anticipate food or drink, to be motivated to eat and drink and to enjoy these activities. In addition, the parents have to be prepared to allow the child to explore and practise these skills.

Self-feeding and the child with cerebral palsy

The child with cerebral palsy is often unable to bring his hands to his mouth. He may have difficulty in grasping or releasing an object. Eye–hand co-ordination may be poor. There is often difficulty in grading (judging) and co-ordinating movement. Involuntary movements interfere with the child's attempts to complete a task. When any child is learning to feed himself we do not expect every mouthful to be a success. It is important to be prepared for mess. Time, patience and encouragement will be important in motivating both the child and the helper.

The Practical Management of Eating & Drinking Difficulties in Children

Appropriate seating will be a necessity. Initially it might be more realistic to provide a stable position for the child so that he can focus his efforts on the more complex tasks of eating or drinking and self-feeding. Remember that the child is normally able to chew before self-feeding develops. Whilst independence is important, it is possible that early emphasis on self-feeding will actually make it more difficult for the child to learn to eat or drink as efficiently as possible. It is obviously important that children do develop as much independence as possible in the long term, but it is worth considering that *improving oral skills before focusing on self-feeding may actually lead to a better future pattern.*

A physiotherapist or occupational therapist will be able to advise on how to help the child become more independent. It is important to discuss this with the speech and language therapist to ensure that the most appropriate strategy is adopted. Information regarding cutlery, crockery and aids to independent eating and so on should be available from a physiotherapist or occupational therapist. (*See Appendix I.*)

Where a child has a visual impairment, a teacher of the visually impaired should also be involved in developing the child's independence in eating and drinking.

'More than a mealtime'

Children normally become involved in food shopping and preparation as a matter of course. They learn about different colours, quantity and so on while going around a supermarket. They acquire vocabulary. They learn where different foods are stored in the home, and watch adults preparing meals and clearing up afterwards. As they grow older they become more involved, helping to stir and taste cake mixtures, and help with washing up. These routine events provide valuable learning experiences.

It may be very difficult to involve a child with special needs in such everyday activities. They can, however, be of enormous benefit; for example, the child may enjoy helping to prepare food for other people although he may be unable to eat it himself. This allows the child to see foods as a source of pleasure and not one of anxiety or boredom. Do try to involve children in food preparation whenever it is safe and possible to do so.

This chapter has examined many ways in which children may be helped to eat and drink more efficiently. There is a vast difference between feeding someone just in order to nourish him and the use of therapeutic eating and drinking, which aims to improve the quality of those activities. *A therapeutic approach can lead to progress in many aspects of development, such as motor skills, communication and self-esteem.*

CHAPTER EIGHT

NUTRITION

INTRODUCTION

When a child has difficulty in eating or drinking the focus of attention may be on how much the child takes rather than on the nutritional value of what is being given. As with any child, a healthy, well balanced diet is important for the child with cerebral palsy. However, refusal to take particular textures and tastes, negative reactions to drinking and so on may lead to justifiable concern regarding the child's nutrition and in particular his weight.

Whenever possible, referral to a dietician who is a specialist in the field of nutrition is strongly recommended. Dieticians are able to analyse food and fluid intake, measure this against an individual's needs and thus provide many practical suggestions on diet to promote optimum growth and enable good health to be maintained. Typical recommendations cover areas such as the use of supplements to increase calorific intake and dealing with the problem of constipation. Children require a combination of foods in order to thrive. The following table lists nutrients, gives some of their sources and explains their function.

THE SOURCE AND FUNCTION OF NUTRIENTS		
Nutrient	*Sources*	*Function*
Protein	**Animal protein:** meat, poultry, fish, eggs, milk, yogurt, cheese **Vegetable protein:** pulses such as lentils, nuts, wholegrain cereals and breads, wheatgerm, tofu (soya bean curd)	Essential for growth, repair of body cells, blood formation, bone development, protection against infection

THE SOURCE AND FUNCTION OF NUTRIENTS		
Nutrient	*Sources*	*Function*
Carbohydrates	**Starch sources:** cereals, wholemeal flours, bread, pulses (such as lentils), potatoes **Sugar sources:** fresh and dried fruits, root vegetables, honey, pasta, sugar (sugar intake should be restricted)	Supplies energy which spares protein for its many other essential functions Major energy provider in the diet
Fibre	Wholegrain cereals, pulses such as chick peas, baked beans, nuts, seeds, dried and fresh fruits, such as bananas, vegetables	Necessary for proper functioning of the digestive tract, but *must be used with care in infant diets*
Fat	**Saturated fat:** butter, cream, whole milk, cheeses, egg yolk, hard fats, animal fats, some margarines **Unsaturated and polyunsaturated fat:** fish oils, some nuts and seeds, oils from nuts, seeds and grains, soft margarines	A useful source of energy. Polyunsaturated fats are essential nutrients and may lower the blood cholesterol level

Nutrient	Sources	Function
Fat-soluble vitamins		
Vitamin A	Oily fish, fish liver oils, liver, egg yolk, dairy produce, fortified margarine. Carotene is converted to Vitamin A in the body and is supplied by carrots, tomatoes, all green and some yellow vegetables, dried apricots, swede, peas, prunes	Essential for proper function of eyesight. Important for normal growth and health of skin, hair and nails. Increases resistance to infection
Vitamin D	Oily fish, fish liver oils, egg yolk, dairy fats, fortified margarine	Formed in the body by the action of direct sunlight on the skin and essential for absorption of calcium required for bones and teeth. Absence of vitamin D can result in rickets
Vitamin E	Wheat, rice and oatgerms, wholegrain cereals, green leafy vegetables, nuts, seeds, pulses, soya flour, cold pressed vegetable oils	Improves general vitality. Important for integrity of cell structure and function of heart and muscles
Vitamin K	Green leafy vegetables, tomatoes, liver, egg yolk, soya bean oil, bananas	Essential for blood clotting to to prevent excess blood loss after injury
Water-soluble vitamins		
B group B1 Thiamin	Wholegrain cereals, especially cereal germs, brewer's yeast, yeast extracts, nuts and sesame seeds (available in paste form called tahini), green leafy vegetables, pulses, meat, egg yolk, malt extract	Essential for the proper metabolism of starch and sugars. Important for the health of the skin, hair, muscles, nerves, brain, eyes and blood

Nutrient	Sources	Function
B2 Riboflavin	Wholegrain cereals, brewer's yeast, nuts, seeds, fish, meat, dairy produce, eggs, potatoes, green leafy vegatables, pulses, malt extract	Important for the health of the skin, hair, muscles, nerves, brain, eyes and blood
B3 Niacin	Wholegrain cereals, brewer's yeast, nuts, seeds, meat, fish, pulses, green leafy vegetables, mushrooms, dried apricots, malt extract	Important for the health of the skin, hair, muscles, nerves, brain, eyes and blood
B6 Pyridoxin	Wholegrain cereals, wheatgerm, fish, pulses, soya flour, liver, chicken, walnuts, peanuts, bananas, avocado pears, malt extract	Important for the health of the skin, hair, muscles, nerves, brain, eyes and blood
Vitamin B12	Liver, dairy food, fortified foods, malt and yeast extracts. The best sources are found in animal foods	Essential for red blood cell formation and integrity of nerve cells. Diets excluding all animal produce may need dietary supplements of vitamin B12
Folic acid	Wholegrain cereals, pulses, soya flour, green leafy vegetables, mushrooms, egg yolk, oranges, brewer's yeast, potatoes, cow's milk, avocado pears	Essential for blood formation. Deficiency of this vitamin causes anaemia
Vitamin C (Ascorbic acid)	Fresh fruit, especially berries and citrus fruits, green leafy vegetables, tomatoes, potatoes, melons	Increases resistance to infection. Encourages tissue repair and normal growth. Important for the absorption of iron.

Nutrient	Sources	Function
Minerals		
Calcium	Sesame seeds, cheeses, milk, blackstrap molasses, almonds, green leafy vegetables, pulses, soya flour, yogurt, dried fruit, brewer's yeast, tinned salmon, sardines, tofu (soya bean curd)	Needed for building bones and teeth. Involved in blood clotting. Important for heart function and health of the skin. See vitamin D function
Iron	Brewer's yeast, blackstrap molasses, liver, red meats, sesame seeds, wholegrain cereals, green leafy vegetables, dried fruits, pulses, soya flour, egg yolk, sardines, almonds, tofu (soya bean curd)	Essential for blood and muscle formation. The absorption of iron is aided by foods containing vitamin C
Magnesium	Nuts, seeds, wholegrain cereals, dried fruits, soya beans, pulses, brewer's yeast, fruits, vegetables	Required for proper metabolism of carbohydrate. Involved in bone and teeth formation
Phosphate	Usually present with calcium	Required with calcium for formation of bones and teeth
Potassium	Fruits, such as bananas, vegetables, seaweeds, pulses, soya flour, wholegrain cereals, nuts, seeds, brewer's yeast, blackstrap molasses, meat, fish	Essential for growth and the proper function of the heart
Sodium	Table salt, soya sauce, celery, meats, cheese, nuts, egg yolk, dairy produce	Sodium is involved in many of the vital body processes, but salt should not be added to food for babies under 12 months old
Sulphur	Wholegrain cereals, pulses, soya flour, almonds, meat, eggs	Important for the health of the hair and nails

THE SOURCE AND FUNCTION OF NUTRIENTS

Nutrient	Sources	Function
Trace elements		
Zinc	Nuts, seeds, meats, fish, egg yolk, poultry, dairy produce, brewer's yeast, wholegrain cereals, yellow and green vegetables, especially peas, and yellow fruits like mango	A vital component of several enzymes concerned with digestion of carbohydrate and protein. Essential for normal growth/healing
Iodine	Sea foods, seaweed, fish liver oils, pulses, soya flour, green vegetables, salt, garlic	Essential for proper metabolism, controlled by the thyroid gland, which requires iodine for formation of thyroid hormone
Manganese	Wholegrain cereals, rice, wheat and oat germs, nuts, vegetables, pulses, soya flour, liver, berries	Essential for the utilization of vitamin B1. Helps reproduction and lactation
Selenium	Wholegrain cereals, rice, wheat and oat germs, nuts, vegetables, pulses, soya flour, liver, berries	Metabolic processes and function

If a child is unable to take certain foods, it may be necessarry to consider giving a vitamin and/ or mineral supplement. This should be discussed with the doctor or dietician.

Safety note: Nuts should only be given if they are finely ground or in a smooth paste form, as in peanut butter.

INTRODUCING SOLID FOOD

Unless there is a good medical reason for not doing so, try to introduce semi-solids at the usual time, which is from about four months. If weaning is delayed, it may be more difficult for the child with cerebral palsy to adapt to the changes involved. If a baby is taking milk well from breast or bottle and does not readily accept semi-solids, it is easy not to persevere. However, it is *strongly recommended* that semi-solids are offered slowly and carefully to enable the child to *learn how to deal with them*. Whilst weaning may take a longer time than usual, it is an important stage in development which will help pave the way for later chewing skills and speech production. Health visitors are usually able to advise on the types of food and dietary requirements appropriate to the baby or child's age. Many health authorities publish helpful booklets, as do most of the baby food manufacturers. Your local hospital's dietetic department may also be able to provide useful information.

Many children with cerebral palsy find eating smooth semi-solids easier than drinking milk. The thicker consistency is easier to control and can stimulate more mature tongue and lip movements. Try to avoid bottle-feeding for any longer than is necessary, but not at the expense of adequate fluid intake. Remember to respect cultural differences. Prolonged sucking may lead to later feeding problems. As the baby grows older, the emotional attachment to a bottle can be very difficult to break. Extra time spent early on can prevent more long-term difficulties. New foods should be offered when the baby or child is happy and not tired. *Remember to position the baby or child carefully (see Chapter 5)* so that he has the best possible chance of coping well with a new experience.

Babies often appear to spit out their first solids. This is not deliberate. Consider how the baby's tongue moves during sucking — in a forward–backward manner. The baby therefore reacts to the spoon and solids in the same way, resulting in their often being returned to the feeder! Perseverance leads to changes in mouth movements and gradual improvement in taking the food. Only offer *one* new food every few days. This will help establish whether or not any subsequent reactions are due to an allergy to a specific food. *Never force* babies to accept food: this is likely to make them refuse it even more vigorously the next time.

Most babies do not need to be weaned before four months of age (*see Chapter 2 for further details*). Milk is the most important food for a baby throughout the first year of life. This, possibly with the addition of a vitamin supplement and boiled water, is all that is required for the first four to six months of life. *Do not add cereals or other food to bottle feeds*.

The first foods offered are frequently a *smooth, thin* fruit or vegetable purée or a baby rice. Offer half to one teaspoon *before* the milk feed. *Do not add salt or sugar to the food*. Fruit such as stewed, peeled eating apples, pears, apricots and pitted prunes can be liquidized. Seeded fruit such as raspberries should not be used as the seeds are too difficult for babies to eat safely. Vegetables such as boiled carrots, parsnips, swede, potatoes, peas (fresh or frozen) can be liquidized. Tomatoes may be used as long as the seeds and skin have been removed. A useful tip is to liquidize batches of individual fruit or vegetables and freeze in ice cube trays, defrosting and using as required.

WAYS TO INCREASE THE VARIETY OF TEXTURES AND TASTES YOU CAN OFFER THE CHILD

Offer *baby cereals*, starting with baby rice *only* once a day. *Avoid rusk and other wheat cereals until the age of six months* in case the baby has an intolerance of wheat protein (gluten). Most manufactured baby foods indicate whether or not they are gluten-free on the packaging. *Home-made vegetable soup* may be liquidized to form a thick purée. Do not add salt or excess seasoning. *Commercial baby foods* can be useful, but it is important to follow the instructions given with the product. To make the food more nutritious it can be made up with formula milk instead of water. You can thicken food using items such as *Ready Brek*, crumbled *Weetabix*, instant mashed potato flakes or powder, sponge cake or breadcrumbs. Note that it is often advised to keep babies off any gluten until 12 months of age. As babies eat more solids, they will become thirsty. Offer cooled boiled water or well diluted unsweetened fruit juice between meals, particularly in warm weather. However, do not give them too close to meals, otherwise the baby will not want to take the more nutritionally sound food.

Fruit squashes containing sugar and colourings are unsuitable. Breast or formula milk should be used until the child is one year old. Cow's milk may then be used as a replacement unless otherwise recommended. See Chapter 7 for information on chewing skills. *Remember that all equipment used for preparing, cooking and sieving or liquidizing food for young babies should be thoroughly washed, rinsed and dried.*

NUTRITIONAL PROBLEMS THAT MAY BE SEEN IN CHILDREN WITH CEREBRAL PALSY

Inadequate weight gain

Dieticians are the best people to consult regarding increasing calorific intake. Referral to your local dietetic department can be made by your general practitioner. The following suggestions may be useful.

Use of supplements

Some, such as *Ensure*, *Fresubin*, *Paediasure* and *Enrich*, provide energy and protein. Expert advice is required before introducing these products because the protein levels in them are too high for some age groups. Other supplements such as *Hycal*, *Maxijul*,

Duocal and *Liquigen* provide just energy. Some supplements, including *Enrich* and *Fresubin* plus fibre, have fibre added.

Other ways to increase calories include the following:

◆ Add cream to puddings, potato, porridge and so on.
◆ Add butter or margarine to vegetables.
◆ Fry food whenever possible.
◆ Melt chocolate into puddings and milk drinks.
◆ Add cheese to sauces and potato.
◆ Add smooth peanut butter to vegetables.
◆ Include pastry where suitable.
◆ Use fortified milk. This is made by adding two tablespoons of skimmed milk powder to a pint of whole milk. (This is for use by older children.)
◆ Use snacks. (*Caution:* a child may become 'full up' and refuse meals if these are given too frequently.)
◆ Use whole milk yogurts, fromage frais.
◆ Use cheeses with a high fat content, such as cream cheese and Cheddar.

Healthy eating principles are not always appropriate for the child with cerebral palsy. However, your dietician can help you if you are concerned about the use of fats or sugar.

The Practical Management of Eating & Drinking Difficulties in Children

Inadequate fluid intake

The following chart is a guide to the daily fluid requirements of babies and children.

AGE	FLUID/KG BODY WEIGHT
Baby (less than 12 months)	120–150 ml/kg body weight
1–2 years	120 ml/kg body weight
2 years	100 ml/kg body weight
3–6 years	90 ml/kg body weight
7–8 years	70 ml/kg body weight
9–11 years	65 ml/kg body weight
11 years	40–60 ml/kg body weight
11–14 years	55 ml/kg body weight
14–18 years	50 ml/kg body weight

This may help parents or carers to gauge the adequacy of fluid intake of their children. However, a dietician is able to provide a more accurate assessment by taking account of the fluid content of fruit, vegetables and other foods.

Suggestions for increasing fluid intake

Offer *thick drinks*, as these are often easier to manage than regular squashes and milk. (*See Chapter 7.*) The following drinks should be diluted with water or milk and mixed to a uniform consistency:

Milk-based drinks — yogurt, fromage frais; liquidized melted ice cream or milk and fruit such as banana; unset jelly made with milk and water; custard; semolina; cheese sauce;

Water-based drinks — tomato juice; unset jelly made with water; diluted fruit and vegetable purées; liquidized soup.

Other thick drinks include: soya-based desserts such as *Provamel* (available from health food shops). (*See Appendix II for further ideas.*)

The following agents can be used to thicken fluids.

Thixo-D is made from corn and maize starch and is mixed into either hot or cold liquids. It should be used with caution for children under one year. It is available on prescription and should only be used under the supervision of a doctor or dietician.

Carobel is made from carob beans. It should be added to (not very hot) liquid then mixed vigorously — using a blender helps to prevent lumps. The final consistency should be thick and smooth. It tends to thicken further on standing. It may be available on prescription at the general practitioner's discretion.

Nestargel has to be boiled first. It becomes thicker on standing, so should be used in small quantities. This is available on prescription at the discretion of the general practitioner.

Thick 'n' Easy is a prescribable thickener which has a high sodium content. Its use should be carefully monitored.

Vitaquick is a prescribable thickener which has the advantage of not thickening on standing.

Cornflour and water: mix as for everyday cooking.

Potato: dried or soft-boiled — can be added to soups.

Constipation

This is often a problem in children with cerebral palsy, resulting from lack of movement, poor fluid intake, lack of dietary fibre, or other physiological factors. It also compounds the problem of being underweight as the child is unable to take more food if the gut is 'blocked'. Dealing with the problem as soon as possible is recommended.

Lack of movement

A physiotherapist may be able to suggest exercises and/or abdominal massage to increase abdominal movement. Indeed, standing can be effective, as gravity helps the child to pass the motion. Standing may be particularly helpful for children with low muscle tone.

Poor fluid intake

Increasing fluid intake (see previous section) is of particular importance as fibre-containing foods require fluid to absorb. You should *always increase fluid intake when fibre intake is increased*.

Lack of dietary fibre

The following foods are good sources of fibre:

◆ Wholemeal bread.
◆ Wholegrain breakfast cereals, *Weetabix*, *Ready Brek* and so on.
◆ Dried fruit and their juices, such as diluted prune juice (from health food shops).
◆ Fresh fruit such as bananas.
◆ Pulses, lentil soup, humus.
◆ Vegetables such as carrots.
◆ Wholewheat pasta and brown rice.
◆ Nuts — use smooth nut butter, such as peanut and almond, in vegetables, soups and sauces. *These are not suitable for young children.*
◆ Fruit juices.
◆ Unprocessed bran can be added to gravy and puréed food — this should *only be done after discussion with a dietician and needs to be carefully supervised.*

The following recipe has been found helpful in easing constipation (please note that recommended quantities are approximate and will vary according to the child's age and weight).
Liquidize the following:

One 300g tin prunes (pitted) and the juice
300 ml water
Three large ripe bananas
225g dried fruit, such as raisins, apricots, peaches previously soaked in the 300 ml water

This makes 1000 ml. Extra water may be added to this mixture if required. Divide into 40 portions (it freezes well in, for example, ice cube trays). Give one portion per day at one or more meals.

Do not be tempted to increase the 'dose' too soon if the child has not passed a motion. It takes up to four days for food to pass through the digestive system but varies with the individual, so wait for that time before deciding whether or not to increase the 'dose'. If you do give more, increase by no more than an extra tablespoon in one day.

Some people find that the cultures contained in 'live' yogurt have a laxative effect. Warm rather than cool drinks may be helpful.

Dental decay

See Chapter 9 on dental hygiene.

Specific nutritional deficiencies

These may include such problems as inadequate iron or vitamin B12 intake. Specialist advice should be sought. Check with a dietician or health visitor regarding vitamin supplements.

Allergies

A small percentage of babies or children are unable to tolerate particular foods, such as cow's milk, eggs, wheat and additives such as E102 — Tartrazine. Specialist advice should be sought before commencing a strict diet, as serious nutritional deficiencies can develop.

Obesity

This is not a frequent problem in children with cerebral palsy but it should be remembered that an overweight child will have more difficulty both in moving and in being moved by adults. It is easier to prevent obesity than to treat it.

A word about vegetarian diets

An increasing number of families are vegetarian. In addition, many children with cerebral palsy have difficulty eating meat and, to a lesser extent, fish. Children do not need to eat meat and fish provided other sources of protein are available. However, they should ideally take two servings of pulses every day to ensure an adequate iron intake if meat and fish are excluded from their diet. Refer to the table at the beginning of the chapter for further details on sources of protein and iron.

With vegan diets, supplements of Vitamin B12 and possibly iron may be required. A calcium-enriched soya milk is recommended for the vegan child. Careful management of nutritional intake will be required.

NON-ORAL FEEDING

In some cases a baby or child will experience such difficulty in eating or drinking that he does not take in adequate nourishment. It is not uncommon for feeding to take several hours and this presents both physical and emotional problems for the child and his feeder. Meals may seem to be never-ending and often become battlegrounds where no one wins. They may be a constant source of stress. A baby or child may experience such problems during feeding that he coughs, splutters and chokes. Vomiting may occur routinely. All these factors may contribute to the decision to use a tube for feeding. Many parents understandably become distressed at the thought of their child being fed by tube, but it is hoped that the following information will help people to understand the role of tube-feeding in *therapy* as well as in providing adequate nutrition.

Attitudes to tube-feeding vary greatly. This applies equally to the opinions of parents, doctors and other professional staff. Parents and therapists may see it as indicating a failure to manage oral feeding. Some people may view tube-feeding as a permanent means of supplying nutrition to a baby or child. This is not always the case. However, we should consider the possible effects on the baby or child of continued feeding by mouth where this presents difficulties.

1 A great deal of time and energy is spent trying to feed the child, with little success.
2 The situation is often very stressful for the child and feeder.
3 The child may associate unpleasant or even painful experiences with feeding, especially if there are problems such as a bite reflex, choking, dental pain and constipation, or if tubes required for feeding or suctioning are frequently passed. In addition, the child may *not* experience any pleasant oral experiences to counteract the negative sensations and hence the problem may worsen. Remember that babies normally start to put their fingers, toys and later toes to their mouth from about four months of age — this provides a wide range of largely pleasurable stimulation.
4 The child may be receiving inadequate amounts of food or fluid.
5 Feeding may be *potentially dangerous* if the child is aspirating (food or fluid entering the airway).
6 The child is likely to be using abnormal patterns of movement rather than developing more normal co-ordination of tongue, lips and jaw. These may be associated with poor positioning, which again reinforces undesirable movement.
7 Feeding may continue to be very messy.
8 Mealtimes may be isolated to meet the child's special needs in terms of seating and so on.
9 The child may have gastro-oesophageal reflux. The mechanism of gastro-oesophageal reflux is not clearly understood. One of the explanations is that the muscle fibres of the diaphragm, which function as a sphincter at the lower end of the oesophagus (gullet), fail to act in a co-ordinated manner, which allows backward flow of stomach contents back up to the oesophagus and pharynx. If the child with cerebral palsy has

increased muscle tone in the abdominal muscles this will encourage reflux. Hip flexion will have a similar effect, therefore careful positioning after meals is very important. It is unpleasant and the acid irritation can reduce the child's desire for food. Drugs may be helpful, for example Cisapride, which encourages the mechanism by which the oesophagus empties.

The two most routinely used methods of non-oral feeding are via a nasogastric or gastrostomy tube.

Nasogastric tube

A thin catheter (tube) is inserted into one nostril and then passed over the back of the soft palate, down behind the tongue into the oesophagus (gullet) and then into the stomach. The catheter has to be changed regularly. Silk tubes are now available which will last three months or more. They are slightly fiddly to put in, but most people can be taught how to manage them.

Gastrostomy

This involves the insertion of a tube directly into the stomach through the abdominal wall. The tube is secured with a plastic button and/or tape onto the child's stomach. Tubes generally need to be replaced every six weeks or so, depending on the choice of tube used. Until recently this operation was performed only under general anaesthetic. A few hospitals have begun using a procedure called percutaneous endoscopic gastrostomy (PEG) which can be performed using a local anaesthetic while the child is sedated. This procedure is increasingly used in the United Kingdom. Results from studies carried out in the past 10 years or so have shown that it is more successful, being quicker, having fewer post-operative complications and involving fewer risks than gastrostomy performed under general anaesthetic.

For both nasogastric and gastrostomy feeding, a sterile feed is used to supply the child's nutrition. The feed may be administered throughout the day and night, or overnight only, depending on the child's nutritional requirements. Whichever method of tube-feeding is employed, a pump is normally used to ensure that the correct volume of food is given during a set period of time. The two methods are compared in the following table.

	NASOGASTRIC TUBE	**GASTROSTOMY**
Appearance	An obvious sign of difficulty in eating may attract unwanted attention, especially in an older child	Not visible unless child is undressed
Ease of removal by child	Babies and children may find it irritating and pull it out	More difficult for baby or child to remove unless undressed
Effect on breathing	One nostril is effectively 'blocked up' by the tube. This is particularly distressing for babies (who normally breathe through their nose) and where a baby or child is trying to eat by mouth and should not therefore be breathing through his mouth simultaneously	No effect
Effect on gag reflex	The gag reflex may become less sensitive in response to the presence of a foreign body. This is especially true where a tube is used long-term	No effect

	NASOGASTRIC TUBE	**GASTROSTOMY**
Effect on feeding by mouth	The child may experience abnormal, often unpleasant sensations because of the presence of the nasogastric tube, although this should not happen if fine-bore tubing is used	Mouth is left 'free'
Emotional effect	Pressure to feed child remains. Focus of attention at mealtimes is the mouth	Pressure on child to eat or drink greatly diminished. The emphasis on the mouth may be reduced
Duration of non-oral feeding	A useful *short-term* (ie, weeks, not months) measure or supplement to oral feeding	Useful where successful oral feeding is unlikely within approximately four–six months
Effect on sensation	Child often develops negative associations in and around the mouth. Hypersensitivity will reinforce abnormal patterns of movement, especially if the tube can only be inserted via one nostril	Child is able to experience pleasant, non-threatening oral sensations, such as sucking a dummy, smelling food, tasting food or liquid, both between and during feeds
Effect on therapy to improve oral feeding	The presence of a nasogastric tube makes this far more difficult, for reasons described earlier, and the problems may worsen	Where the mouth is free of invasive and other unpleasant stimuli, it is much easier to introduce pleasant stimuli to the child in a controlled, non-pressurized manner
Reversibility	Nasogastric tubes can easily be removed	The gastrostomy can be left to close up, just like any stoma (hole). If the tube is removed accidentally, a new one must be inserted as soon as possible

	NASOGASTRIC TUBE	**GASTROSTOMY**
Child's self-image	Child aware of being tube-fed, but can be fed overnight to reduce awareness	Child can be fed during the night using a pump system, so does not see himself as being tube-fed
Effect on posture/movement	The child is likely to become more hypersensitive and abnormal patterns of movement may increase	Child has to be positioned to avoid abdominal discomfort
Communication	Often difficult because of the stressful nature of the experience	Less pressure and more time can provide a more conducive atmosphere in which better communication between feeder and child can be established
Ease of use	No risk of general anaesthetic. Most parents can be taught to pass tubes at home, although a few find it extremely difficult and never manage it	Risk of general anaesthetic where one is used. Most parents can be taught to manage tube-feeding and to replace tubes at home

In general I would recommend gastrostomy as the feeding method of choice where a child is likely to be unable to feed adequately by mouth for at least four to six months. However, feeding therapy should be instigated and attempts at oral feeding made as recommended by the team caring for the child. This will require time and skilled management. Oral feeding should not be carried out if it is unsafe to do so.

It is essential that the child's nutritional requirements are considered when planning therapy aims and strategies.

CHAPTER NINE

DENTAL

HYGIENE

INTRODUCTION

As with any child, good dental care is an important part of daily routine activities. Babies and children who have difficulties in eating and drinking require particular attention for the following reasons:

1 Breathing through the mouth leads to dryness of the front gums, which causes irritation and possible bleeding.
2 Some anticonvulsant drugs such as Phenytoin can cause the gums to grow over the teeth. This may occur before the teeth have erupted fully and needs to be watched vigilantly. It can lead to gums bleeding.
3 The diet may be high in sugars to increase calorie intake. Sugars are known to contribute to dental decay.
4 The use of a soft diet reduces stimulation of the gums and teeth.
5 Hypersensitivity and/or increased muscle tone in and around the mouth may make tooth cleaning and dental treatment difficult. In some cases children have required a general anaesthetic in order to have dental work carried out. Prevention of dental decay is therefore of very great importance, as prevention is preferable to treatment.
6 Dribbling results in a poor supply of saliva being available within the mouth to keep it clean and moist.
7 Dental hygiene provides excellent stimulation, which helps with chewing and saliva control. Such early oral stimulation can lead to increased tolerance of food textures and it is really worth persevering with the activities suggested below.

IMPROVING DENTAL HYGIENE

The following guidelines are designed to improve the baby's/child's dental hygiene.

1 Seek advice from the local or community dental surgeon regarding the use of *fluoride* supplements. These can reduce dental decay by 50 per cent or more. The dentist will be aware of local levels of fluoride in the water supply and advise accordingly.
2 When cleaning a child's teeth, use a fluoride toothpaste. If the child swallows it, ask the dentist if supplements are still required. *Note*: it is possible to take in too much fluoride, but this does not become obvious until the second teeth have erupted. They will appear mottled. This should not put people off using fluoride supplements. However, it does illustrate the need to check details with the dentist. A health visitor may also be able to advise.
3 Leaflets on dental care may be available from a local dentist or health visitor.
4 Introduce *gum massage* even before the first tooth has come through (see below). *Teeth need gums.* Gums provide the foundation within which the teeth form. If the gums become unhealthy and swollen and start to bleed, they are unable to support the teeth.

CLEANING THE GUMS

When massaging one's own baby's gums, most practitioners would not suggest wearing protective gloves (like those worn by dentists). However, most people working with other people's children or babies are either obliged or encouraged to use such garments. This is to protect both parties from possible infection. Where gloves are not worn, scrupulous hand washing is advisable. Wrapping a little gauze or muslin around the finger may be helpful, although it should be wetted before placement in the child's mouth as this is more comfortable. Warm water (previously boiled for babies) is often best as it does not have any taste or smell which could stimulate excessive saliva production. Milk (breast milk where this is being given) can also be used for this purpose. Given relative hand sizes, most women would be advised to use their little finger (or index finger with children over five years of age) and men should generally use their little finger.

Positioning the baby or child

As for feeding, it is important that the child is comfortable with his head upright and in mid-line (symmetrical alignment) with an elongated back of neck and slightly tucked in chin. Sitting on the adult's lap is acceptable if guidelines described in Chapter 5, on positioning, are followed. Gum massage should be pleasurable and should not be continued if the child shows any discomfort or distress.

Procedure

Proceed as described in Chapter 7. (See also Figures 12a–12c.) Start by rolling your finger inside the top lip, slightly off centre. Firmly rub the upper gums along the line of the jaw on one side, backward and forward up to three times; that is, massaging a quarter of the mouth. Repeat along the upper gums of the other side, then the other side's lower gums, then the remaining side's lower gums.

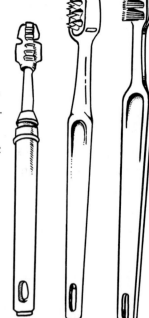

Figure 26 *Dental training set for stimulating gums and teeth*

It is important to give the child *time* to swallow after each section has been stimulated, or less often if appropriate. Keep the mouth as closed as possible during this activity. Providing oral control, as described in Chapter 7, may be helpful. There are now some special products available designed to stimulate gums. (See *Dental Training in Appendix I* and Figure 26.) Use these as described above and/or to massage gums in small circular movements.

CLEANING THE TEETH

A small, narrow-headed, soft–medium-bristle or nylon toothbrush can be introduced as soon as the first tooth has erupted, as long as it is tolerated by the baby. Continue to use a finger if a brush causes negative reactions such as crying or turning away. If the baby dislikes the brush, consider if it is too long, wide and so on before stopping its use.

Some children with cerebral palsy have a small head and mouth and may require a small toothbrush, even at school age. Toothpaste should not be used with very young children who swallow it in excessive quantities or who dislike it. When toothpaste is used, a pea-sized amount is adequate.

Position

The baby or child should be well supported with his head in mid-line (symmetrical alignment) and upright as for feeding. The back of his neck should be elongated with a slightly tucked in chin. An older child should sit opposite a basin or bowl to allow him to rinse and spit out excess water. The adult can sit to his side to provide support to head and jaw as necessary.

Procedure

The brush is used in a similar pattern to gum massage, starting on the side which is best tolerated by the child. Roll the head of the brush under the top lip so that the bristles do not touch outside the mouth (see Figures 27a and 27b) causing excessive stimulation. Treat the mouth in four sections (see Figure 27c) as for gum massage. Move the brush as high up as possible on the top teeth and as low down as possible on the lower teeth. Keep the mouth as closed as possible during this activity. (See 'Oral Control', pages 56–7.)

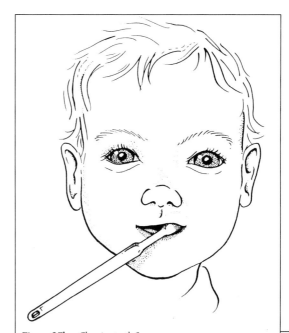

Figure 27b   *Cleaning teeth 2*
Note: Continue rolling toothbrush to this position.

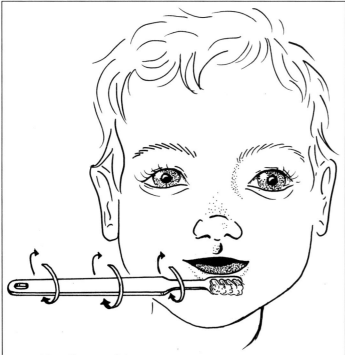

Figure 27a   *Cleaning teeth 1*
Note: Roll the head of the toothbrush under the top lip, bristles facing outwards, then down.

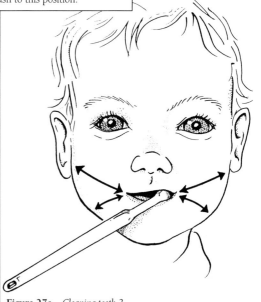

Figure 27c   *Cleaning teeth 3*
Note: Brush teeth in direction of arrows.

The Practical Management of Eating & Drinking Difficulties in Children

Move along the teeth and back to the starting point using a downward movement for the top teeth and an upward movement for the lower teeth. When you have completed all four sections give the child a sip of water (if possible) and encourage spitting out by bringing the child's cheeks in to purse the lips (see Figure 28).

Repeat the sequence of tooth brushing along the inside of the teeth. The movement will be vertical at the front of

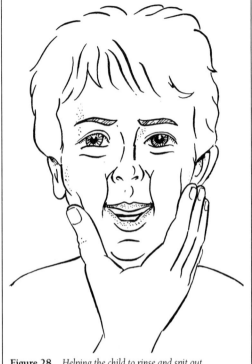

Figure 28   *Helping the child to rinse and spit out*
Note: Bring the child's cheeks forward to purse the lips.

the mouth, becoming diagonal at the back (see Figure 29). Remove the brush and rinse as before.

Finally, brush the biting surfaces of the molars and premolars (chewing teeth) in the same sequence, moving along the line of the teeth. Remove the brush and rinse as before.

Remember that this activity is stimulatory and saliva production may be increased. Appropriate support to head, jaw and/or mouth should therefore be provided and *time* given for the child to swallow. Some children may only tolerate brushing the outside of the teeth at first. Practising this sequence should gradually enable you to put the brush inside the mouth. Start off centre to reduce the incidence of a bite reflex. Do not present the brush too far back at the sides, as this may cause gagging.

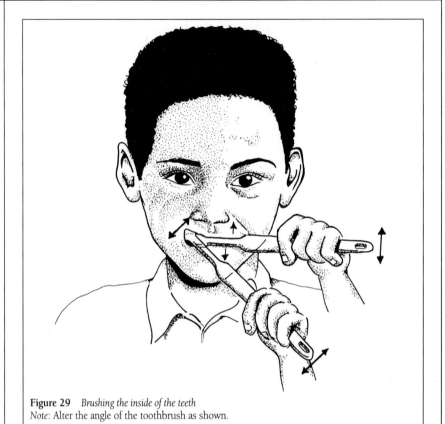

Figure 29   *Brushing the inside of the teeth*
Note: Alter the angle of the toothbrush as shown.

Electric toothbrushes

From the age of three years or so, an electric toothbrush can be very useful. Use it without the power switched on until you and the child feel comfortable with it. Use it on yourself to feel how much pressure is comfortable. Practise using it on adults and children who do not have eating or drinking difficulties, so that they can let you know how it feels and how you might need to alter your technique.

As well as stimulating the gums and teeth, an electric toothbrush may enable a child with cerebral palsy to clean his teeth independently.

FREQUENCY OF TOOTH CLEANING

Ideally, the child's teeth should be cleaned after each meal, snack or sweet drink. Where this is not possible, do try to get the child used to dental care at least after breakfast and before bedtime.

Try to take the child along to your own dental check-ups to familiarize him with the surgery and staff. Find out about local services. Some health authorities employ dentists who specialize in treating children with special needs.

There is a difference between routine teeth cleaning and the careful, thorough 'therapeutic toothbrushing' described here. *The long-term benefits of therapeutic toothbrushing make it a worthwhile and important part of the child's day.*

CHAPTER TEN

THE MANAGEMENT OF DRIBBLING

INTRODUCTION

Children learn to swallow their saliva as they acquire physical skills, notably head and trunk control. A baby who has begun to dribble less may start to do so more when acquiring new skills such as walking or running. Teething may also increase dribbling, though this is temporary. In normal development, control of dribbling is learnt automatically.

◆ PRACTICAL EXERCISE 14

This is to make you aware of how it feels to swallow to command.

1 I want you to swallow now!

How does it feel to swallow when told to do so? Most people find this difficult.

2 Now swallow twice in succession.

Whilst you will have managed one swallow, the second swallow would have been impossible until you had produced more saliva. We are unable to swallow unless we have *something* to swallow.

SALIVA AND ITS FUNCTIONS

Saliva is mainly produced by three pairs of salivary glands. This occurs on an involuntary basis, although we can deliberately make ourselves produce saliva by, for example, thinking of food. Saliva has seven main functions:

1 It protects the teeth and gums.
2 It prepares food for chewing and swallowing.
3 It initiates the digestion of carbohydrates.

4 It lubricates the tongue and lips during speech.
5 It assists with oral hygiene by cleaning the mouth.
6 It regulates acidity within the mouth and gut.
7 It facilitates tasting — we can only taste when food is in solution.

The control of saliva is therefore not only important because dribbling is messy and socially unacceptable, but also because its presence in the mouth is necessary.

DIFFICULTIES WITH SALIVA CONTROL

It is estimated that an adult produces one to one and a half litres of saliva in 24 hours, resulting in 1,000 to 2,000 swallows per day. Amounts vary from person to person. Individuals have also been shown to produce different amounts under various circumstances, for example as a side-effect of drugs. Saliva control largely depends on trunk stability and good head control, as well as on the ability to be aware of the need to swallow. Complex co-ordination of swallowing and breathing is required.

As children with cerebral palsy have difficulty with co-ordination and fine selective movements, it is not surprising that dribbling is a common problem. They may also have sensory problems so that they are unaware of the need to swallow. A wet chin may feel 'normal'.

Dribbling results in many problems including:

◆ loss of fluid,
◆ sore mouth,
◆ wet, dirty clothes,
◆ discomfort of a dry mouth,
◆ more difficult speech,
◆ more difficult eating,
◆ unhealthy mouth, leading to bad breath and gum or dental problems,
◆ wet furniture, books, toys and so on,
◆ social unacceptability,
◆ embarrassment.

The ability of children to control their own saliva will vary according to many factors, including positioning, concentration, fatigue, health, mood, motivation and drugs taken.

MANAGEMENT OF SALIVA CONTROL

Position

We need to be able to help children from as early an age as possible. Our handling of babies and children should provide the support required to enable them to experience what it is like to have an upright head with lips together. Should the child have difficulty breathing in this situation, medical advice or a physiotherapist's opinion should be sought. (A physiotherapist may be able to offer advice regarding lip closure and breath control through the use of hydrotherapy and swimming for children with cerebral palsy.)

Remember that some children may be unable to breathe through their nose, for example if they are 'blocked up', so that holding their mouth closed is inappropriate.

Children should be well supported and upright, with an elongated back of the neck. Where necessary, oral control can be

given to provide jaw stability, as described in Chapter 7. There should not be any pressure on the child to swallow. He should be calm and relaxed. Watching video tapes, listening to audio tapes, or listening to the adult singing or telling a story may be helpful. It is important not to continue if the child becomes distressed, or he will struggle when the activity is subsequently repeated. Short, frequent periods of such handling help the child to experience more normal saliva control. As children acquire improved head control and jaw stability, we can expect more spontaneous carry-over; that is, they start to control their saliva in a more automatic manner. However, regression is to be expected when children are engaged in activities requiring concentration and manipulation. Where head control remains poor, it may be unrealistic to expect children to master saliva control independently. *Good positioning is crucial* to allow children to have as much control as possible.

Wiping mouths

When a child's mouth is very wet, it is necessary to dry it. However, the way in which this is done is important, as it can help or hinder progress.

Do nots

1 Do not push the child's head back when wiping the mouth.
2 Do not wipe the mouth *unless it is necessary*.
3 Do not *suddenly* wipe the mouth.
4 Do not wipe it *without* letting the child see (or feel a tactile cue) that the cloth is approaching.
5 Do not use a large piece of flannel, tissue or other material that will touch the sides of the face as well as the mouth. This often increases saliva production, as it provides so much stimulation.
6 Do not wipe the mouth quickly.
7 As far as possible, do not tell the child to swallow. Swallowing is often impossible if the mouth is open and the saliva is on the

chin, bib or table. Being told to swallow may make children self-conscious and anxious.

8 Do not wipe using light movements — they are overstimulating.

Dos

1 Do maintain the child in a good trunk and head position.
2 Do use a *small* tight wodge of absorbent material that will only touch the child's mouth.
3 Do let the child see or feel the approaching cloth.
4 Do approach at a reasonable rate — not too fast or too slow.
5 Do wipe slowly and firmly, using up to three 'pressure dabs', as shown in Figure 30. Start on the side of the mouth which is more easily tolerated by the child.

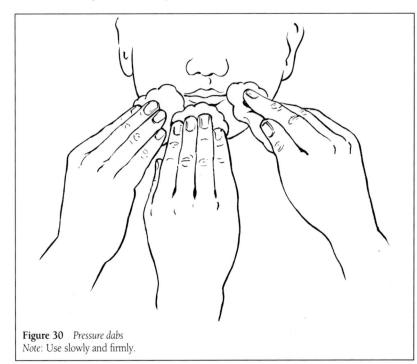

Figure 30 *Pressure dabs*
Note: Use slowly and firmly.

Try it on yourself. If you have done it correctly you should feel the after-effects which encourage you to keep your lips together.

Self-wiping

If children are aware of their dribbling but are unable to prevent it, then being able to keep themselves clean and dry is important. Wearing sweat bands, as used by tennis players, is often very effective, as well as looking acceptable.

Clothing

Specialized designs such as those produced by *Wizzywear* (*see Appendix I*) may be helpful.
Note: where terms such as 'open'/'closed' mouth or 'wet'/'dry' chin are used, it is important to make sure that these are understood by the children. Glove puppets, lip prints (using lipstick), washing and drying hands, crockery and so on can be used to teach these concepts.

Chewing

The development of improved chewing patterns will help with saliva control. (Refer to Chapter 7 for more details.)

Tooth cleaning

The stimulation provided by careful 'therapeutic' toothbrushing can help children learn to control their saliva. (Refer to Chapter 9 for details.)

Behaviour modification

This is appropriate with older children who are motivated to control their own saliva. When children can swallow but do not do so automatically, it may be helpful to use a reward system. Examples of this include stories and timing.

Stories

While the child's mouth is closed, an adult reads a story or plays a tape. As soon as the child's mouth appears to be wet or open, the book is closed or the tape is switched off, but nothing needs to be said. As soon as the child readopts the desired mouth position, the story telling or tape playing recommences, with nothing said. Not using verbal comments is important, as giving instructions puts children under pressure and makes them self-conscious. It does not necessarily help them towards the goal of 'self-awareness': that is, learning to recognize when they need to swallow.

Timing

Some older children will enjoy seeing for how long they can keep themselves dry. They can be timed with a stopwatch and the results may be charted, with stars to indicate progress. This involves self-monitoring and again the adults should avoid commenting until the activity has been completed.

Surgery

Rerouting of salivary gland ducts

This complicated procedure is designed to make it easier for the child to swallow his saliva. Clinical evidence suggests that this is most successful in less affected children from the mid-teens upwards. Specialist advice regarding the feasibility of such an operation should be sought.

Excision of salivary glands

Removing some of the salivary glands has generally been unsuccessful in young children. Whilst there may be a short-term improvement, it has been found that the remaining glands eventually produce extra saliva to compensate for the loss, so that long-term progress is unlikely. Any surgical procedure should be carefully discussed with the team caring for the child.

Drugs

A number of drugs have been used to help reduce dribbling. For example, *Scopoderm TTS* has recently been used with children of five years and older, with some success. It is given transdermally (through the skin) from a patch taped behind the ear. The drug is released slowly over two to three days and the patch is then replaced for as long as the procedure is deemed appropriate. The drug dries up saliva and, whilst it has proved helpful, it does have side-effects, including drying the eyes (a particular problem for contact lens wearers), increasing thirst and causing eczema in response to the plaster used. Currently the same dose is given to all patients. *Scopoderm* is only available on prescription. A range of drugs which are taken by mouth have also been used, with varying degrees of success. These drugs include *Benztropine*. The use of drugs should be fully discussed with the team caring for the child.

Direct oral stimulation

The principle behind this is that sensory input can help to produce a movement pattern; that is, sensory stimulation can result in more effective swallowing of saliva. However, it should be stressed that the child should be well positioned throughout such activities. The feeder's fingers provide such input when a child's mouth is wiped correctly (see above). Pressure applied around the mouth, using small circular movements of the first finger, may be helpful. The child's head should remain upright and in mid-line (symmetrical alignment). (See Figure 31a.)

Oral control should be provided as required. Swallowing can be facilitated using the adult's middle finger beneath the jaw. Move it slowly and rhythmically up and back between the point of the chin and the angle of the neck where the floor of the mouth joins the neck . (See Figure 20.) Downward pressure with the first finger across the child's upper lip may produce a *spontaneous* swallow, as it reinforces elongation of the neck and lip closure. (See Figure 31b.)

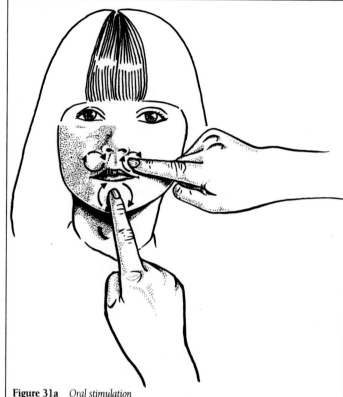

Figure 31a *Oral stimulation*
Note: Small-range circular massage around the mouth may provide helpful stimulation.

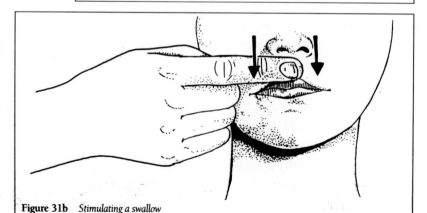

Figure 31b *Stimulating a swallow*
Note: Pressure in a *slightly* downward direction may help to stimulate a swallow.

Procedures described in Chapter 7, on normalizing sensation, and in Chapter 9, on cleaning gums and teeth, are also useful. The child should be well positioned and given time to swallow spontaneously.

Brushing and icing

The use of these stimuli was originally devised by Margaret Rood in North America for use with people who sustained brain damage in adulthood. Strong sensory stimulation was found to produce a physical response. These ideas were adapted for use with children with cerebral palsy. However, the technique remains a controversial area and professionals in the field differ in their attitude towards its use. Many would suggest that neither should be used with children aged under three years, while the nervous system is immature.

Some people recommend the application of ice and brushes to different parts of the face and mouth. Ice is an extremely strong stimulus which can produce adverse effects, for example in a child who is epileptic. If icing is not carried out properly, children may become more sensitive. Anyone contemplating the use of such treatment is strongly advised to ensure that she has been adequately trained in its use.

Training devices

Several devices are available. While they may result in initial success, long-term results are sometimes disappointing. Availability of equipment varies nationally. Items in current use include the *Exeter Lip Sensor*, which reinforces lip closure, bleepers which emit regular noises to remind the child to swallow and palatal training devices. Further information can be obtained from a speech and language therapist.

Travel bands

These wrist-worn bands have a plastic button on them which is designed to stimulate an acupressure point to alleviate the nausea associated with travel sickness. They have never been tested for their effect on saliva production, but some people have reported that, when worn by children who have difficulty in controlling their saliva, the degree of dribbling has lessened. Should their use prove to be effective, it is likely that they would only be appropriate for children with a mild dribbling problem. See Appendix I for details.

Time spent on improving saliva control will also help to develop *more mature eating and drinking patterns*, as well as assisting in good dental care and improved self-image.

CHAPTER ELEVEN

SPECIAL ISSUES REGARDING THE CHILD WITH A VISUAL IMPAIRMENT

Visual impairment can affect both the development of self-feeding and interaction between child and feeder.

◆ PRACTICAL EXERCISE 15

This exercise is to let you experience what it is like to be fed when you are unable to see. You will need someone to help you with this exercise. Take it in turns to feed each other, but ensure that the person being fed is blindfolded. Make sure that you have a variety of foods and drinks available to provide different tastes, textures and temperatures.

1   Use utensils of varying sizes and shapes.

2   Feed each other at various speeds.

3   Compare reactions when a warning that food is approaching is and is not given.

4   Experiment with naming or not naming some foods before presenting them.

Discuss your experiences and identify what was required to make the situation easier and better for the person being fed. Most people find this experience very scary. They feel vulnerable, wary and confused.

The child with visual impairment requires the same opportunities as the normally sighted child to experience different stimuli in the mouth. However, he may need more adult help to make this possible, as inability to see people, food and so on may lower motivation to explore with hands and mouth, even where this is physically possible. In the child with cerebral palsy, meaningful cues to prepare him for these stimuli are crucial, as his reaction may involve an increase in muscle tone and abnormal movement patterns, as well as fear, distress and mistrust. The following suggestions are aimed at improving the whole experience of eating and drinking for the child who has a visual impairment in addition to cerebral palsy.

POSITION

Position the child as well as possible (see Chapter 5) while enabling him to make the best use of any residual vision. A balance needs to be made between the effects of lack of vision or reduced visual field causing abnormal head and trunk posture and abnormal posture and movement attributable to cerebral palsy. A child with a visual impairment without additional problems should always be seated so that his feet are firmly placed on the floor or foot-rest to provide stability and a sense of security.

ENVIRONMENT

1   Ensure that the room is lit to accommodate the child's visual needs. Consider the strength of light, position of light source and that some children may need diffuse lighting. Overhead lighting may encourage the child to look up and backwards. Bright sunlight, particularly through venetian blinds, may irritate the child.

2 Ensure that distracting noises, such as television and radio, are kept to a minimum, as they make it much more difficult for the child to use auditory cues such as voices or a spoon on a plate. Remember that adults filter out many background noises subconsciously. The hum of a machine may not register with the adults in the room but may distract the child. At school, consider where the child is being fed. See Chapter 12 for further information on school mealtimes.

3 Where there is a visual field defect, ensure that the feeder is within the child's visual field. It may be necessary to make compromises when considering the child's visual needs and postural normality. Try to enable the child to have the best function possible.

4 Ensure that the food container and cup are placed within the child's visual field.

5 The use of visual contrasts, such as a white plate or cup on a red non-slip mat, may help the child to locate the food or drink more easily.

FEEDER

1 Trust is a key factor in establishing successful feeding. Where a child is unable to see his feeder well, it is particularly important that the feeder should be a familiar person. In school there should ideally be a consistent feeder, with a deputy to cover for sickness. Such continuity will provide the best possible basis for improvement.

2 The feeder needs to know how the child communicates, and how to respond to these signals in a meaningful way.

COMMUNICATION

1 A carefully planned system of communication is particularly important to enable the child to control his choice of food and drink and the rate at which he is fed. There may be several forms of communication being used, such as the spoken word, signing, objects of reference (where one object represents something else, as with a sponge meaning 'washing') photographs and symbols.

2 Consistent responses are essential. It is unfair to the child if different people respond to a particular gesture in different ways. This may lead to confusion and frustration.

3 There should be clear signals to indicate 'more' or 'no more', 'food' or 'drink'. For example, moving the hands away from the body for 'no more'/'all gone'. See Chapter 3 for further information on communication.

SMELL

We use our sense of smell in many ways. It helps us to anticipate what we are going to eat and drink and it enhances our ability to taste. We make many judgements regarding our likes and dislikes on the basis of how foods smell. We also use smell to recognize people around us, including those who are present at mealtimes.

The child with a visual impairment may be unable to see what is available at mealtimes. He may need to smell what is presented in order to appreciate what is there. It is therefore important to ensure that food smells are always linked to the real item to make it meaningful to the child. For example, if the child smells an orange, then an orange should be available to feel, taste and eat (if safe to do so).

The child can also use his sense of smell to judge where his food is in relation to himself. It can help him to prepare for the approaching spoon or cup both physically (being ready to open his mouth) and emotionally (remaining calm). Individuals vary in their reaction to smells and some caution is needed in their introduction to children to minimize the incidence of strong negative responses, such as withdrawal or crying.

The Practical Management of Eating & Drinking Difficulties in Children

ROUTINE

1 Prepare the child for meals in a specific way, so that he knows what is to follow.
2 Tell the child that it is time to eat or drink.
3 A bib or spoon might be suitable objects of reference to handle. These may be used to help a child anticipate mealtimes if given shortly beforehand.
4 Position the child for meals and tell him what is available. Arrange utensils in a set way. The appropriate places could be marked using a contrasting colour mat or mark.
5 Develop a routine that the child can rely on. For example, once seated, the child is prompted to touch the utensils and food or liquid. The child's face or lips may be touched with a spoon, cup and so on to indicate that food or drink is on its way. If a routine is adopted, the child can learn to anticipate when food or drink will arrive, which decreases startling.
6 Allowing the child to smell his food or drink is important.

UTENSILS

Familiarize the child with feeding equipment through play as he may not be able to see it in everyday use. Choose utensils on the basis of colour, as well as for their role in facilitating better eating and drinking patterns. A child might learn to associate 'drinking time' with the colour of his cup. Present items at an angle which enables the child to use any residual vision.

TACTILE ASPECTS

The child with a severe visual impairment needs to learn about food and drink through touch in the same way as a sighted child. However, what he learns will be of particular value and he will need to continue using this sense, for example to feel how full his cup is or how much is left on a plate and, indeed, to locate the plate. He will need to learn about food textures through handling them to discover which will break, crumble, disintegrate, become sticky and so on.

The child with visual impairment in addition to cerebral palsy may have especial difficulties with tactile defensive behaviour. See page 52.

PRESENTATION

It is helpful to present different foods separately, so that the child can learn to differentiate between colours, such as green peas and orange carrots. This is not possible if foods are mixed together. Similarly textured foods, such as sweetcorn and peas, should not be placed adjacent to each other where a child has poor colour perception.

PREPARATION

The child with a visual impairment should be involved in food shopping and preparation. It is helpful to use a specific supermarket or shop frequently and go around it in a routine way. The child can then learn to associate cold with the ice cream, baking smells with bread, tins with baked beans, and so on.

Putting food away on returning home provides experiences of 'heavy/light', 'cold/not cold', 'breakable/tough' and so on. Keep food and drink in their original containers so that the child can relate them to each other and be able to develop more independence. Most children enjoy being involved in food preparation, for example putting fingers into bowls or being helped to stir using a wooden spoon. Even washing up is fun if you are small, so do try to involve the child in food-related activities as much as possible.

HUNGER AND THIRST

Most of us usually eat and drink in response to feelings of hunger and thirst. Children may not show these feelings if too little time occurs between meals to allow such needs to develop. There are some children, however, who do not experience such feelings and would appear to go happily without sustenance. Some children with a visual impairment fall into this group. It may not be possible for their appetite to be stimulated visually. Such children therefore need to be taught that everyone has to eat or drink. Where there is a visual impairment it will be particularly important to emphasize the social, happy and communicative aspects of mealtimes with these children.

TIME

Children with visual impairments need far longer to go through all processes as they cannot glance around to get swift impressions or knowledge of events. For example, they need to explore the whole plate to know what is for dinner, to dip their fingers into beakers to decide how much drink is there before drinking, and so on. Communication may require extra time and it is very important that these children should not be fed in a hurried way.

SOCIAL ASPECTS

The child needs to learn that other people eat and drink. He can be made aware of who is seated beside him and appreciate that she is drinking and eating too. The happy, sharing aspects of eating and drinking should be emphasized.

INDEPENDENCE

The child with a visual impairment will require specialized help to acquire independence in eating and drinking. It is important that the team of people helping the child discuss his needs and plan appropriate strategies together. Non-slip mats and plate guards may be helpful in preventing food and drink spillage. (*See Appendix I.*)

The child with a visual impairment requires the same opportunities as the normally sighted child. Communication will be of particular importance and the advice of specialist teachers of the visually impaired should be sought.

◆
SPECIAL CONSIDERATIONS RELEVANT TO SCHOOLS

WHILE the subjects covered in this book are relevant to children attending school, there are some issues specific to the needs of pupils and school staff. It is hoped that this chapter will help to address some of the problems which have frequently been discussed with therapists, teachers, nursery nurses, school nurses and welfare staff.

WHERE THE CHILDREN ARE FED

Noise

If you sat in a school dining area and closed your eyes during the mealtime, your initial reaction would probably be "What a noise!" Similar comments are likely to be prompted by watching a video recording of a school meal. The cacophony results from a multitude of sources of sound, such as children crying, dishes falling on the floor, staff talking (or shouting) and perhaps background music. You will probably know what it is like trying to enjoy a meal with someone when the music is on so loud that you cannot hear yourself speak, let alone your companion, or, perhaps, you can hear a drill being used close by, or a neighbour's dog barking. These spoil and may ruin the pleasure of a meal. So what is it like for a child with cerebral palsy? Perhaps he has an additional visual or hearing problem. Some children with impaired hearing find noise or very loud sounds painful and advice should be sought about the use of hearing-aids. How can these children communicate with their feeders or peers if they are unable to differentiate the feeder's voice from surrounding noises? Such conditions may result in an increase in muscle tone (stiffening) and abnormal patterns of movement such as extensor spasms (pushing back). This is particularly undesirable at mealtimes, when such a position makes eating or drinking more difficult and *potentially dangerous*.

Some schools have adopted a policy which insists that all the children are fed together to enhance social development. I would question the value of this for those pupils who are *unable to adapt to the high degree of stimulation* which is unavoidable when a lot of children are being fed together. An alternative, which works well in many schools, is feeding some children in small groups away from the noisy dining room. These can comprise not only those children who are adversely affected by large groups but also some more able pupils. In this way, the social aspects of mealtimes can be maintained while extraneous noise can be diminished. As some of the group will be more able, fewer staff will be required to leave the main dining area.

It has been said that music is played in schools to please the children; however, there are doubts regarding the validity of this claim. Whilst music undoubtedly has a very important role in all schools, I would urge staff to ask for whose benefit it is played during mealtimes. Watching and listening to a video recording of a school meal with music playing is a way of objectively considering its value. I would suggest that most background music is not helpful in a situation which is already noisy and in which many of the children struggle to communicate.

Visual distraction

Schools are usually places filled with colour. Mobiles hang from the ceilings, stained glass window effects abound and walls are covered with murals, paintings and so on. This display is both important and attractive. However, such an array of colour and patterns may make it very difficult for a child with visual problems or high distractibility to cope. It is therefore worth considering the possibility of having *one blank area available* so that such children can be sat facing a calmer, less stimulating expanse.

Interestingly, much of the equipment designed for children with special needs is brightly coloured. Perhaps we ought to reflect on maintaining a balance between helpful and overwhelming visual stimuli. Good visual contrasts, flexible lighting, the direction of light sources and so on should all be considered. Separating small groups of children, as described earlier, may be a viable option where problems such as distractibility exist.

WHEN TO EAT OR DRINK

This may seem to be obvious — children are fed at lunchtime! However, attention should also be paid to snack times such as the mid-morning break. These can provide an invaluable opportunity for practising new approaches to eating and drinking without the pressure to eat and drink that usually accompanies regular meals. They are also very important in helping to provide adequate fluid intake for children, many of whom will find drinking extremely difficult. I suspect that some pupils are reluctant to eat at lunchtime because they are thirsty. The importance of mid-morning or afternoon snacks cannot be overemphasized.

WHO SHOULD FEED THE CHILD

Consistency

At one school I visited, I was told that children were fed by a different person each day. Indeed, on occasions, there was a staff change between courses! It was explained that this policy was designed to prevent overdependence of one child on a specific feeder. Imagine that, from now on, you will eat each meal with someone different. You will not have any idea who your next dining companion will be. After one course that person may suddenly be replaced by someone else. I expect that most people would find this unsettling, so what is it like for the child with cerebral palsy who has difficulty communicating? At the school just mentioned, we discussed this issue for some time, until one teacher said, "Oh, come on, we all swap around because no one wants to have to feed the most difficult children every day." This produced an embarrassed silence. The teacher's point was acknowledged and many people nodded in agreement. However, it was then necessary to look at this issue more closely and explore how to go about changing the system. I am sure that this is not a unique situation.

Many schools have experimented with various schemes to enable the children and their feeders to establish a warm, trusting relationship. One possible option is that, for one term, each child has his own 'main feeder' but a 'deputy' feeds him once a week. Next term the deputy becomes the main feeder and the previous main feeder becomes the main feeder of the child she previously deputized for. And so the chain continues. This continuity is essential if optimal progress is to be seen.

Staff

In schools, the feeders may be teachers, nursery nurses, therapists, welfare staff or other people who are employed specifically to feed the pupils. I was horrified to hear of older pupils feeding younger pupils in one school where staff shortages were severe. Different groups of personnel clearly have different backgrounds, as regards training, experience, expectations and aims for the pupils. Whoever feeds the child needs to see herself as part of a team, which includes the child's parents and, especially with older pupils, the children themselves. Interdisciplinary meetings involving parents and feeders are required at regular intervals. Perhaps one teacher could be the designated liaison person regarding feeding children. She would be responsible for seeking advice, sharing information and so on.

It will be important to discuss each child's needs with the team involved in his care — to listen to and respect each other's opinions and, most importantly of all perhaps, to be open to the possibility of change. Even more important than merely discussing the children is seeing them together, even if this means several people watching a video of the mealtime. This helps to see different points of view. For example, colleagues may all say, "John ate well", but the physiotherapist may mean his head control was good; the speech and language therapist may mean he chewed well; and the person who fed him may mean he ate his fish!

STAFF TRAINING

All the staff involved in the preparation of food or in feeding children should receive some training in the management of eating and drinking difficulties. A description of the content of such a course falls outside the scope of this book, but I would urge all staff to make use of the skills of their therapists. Where therapists do not attend schools on a regular basis, I would nevertheless suggest requesting some training input.

This training should not be restricted to teachers. All the staff who feed children are important people who need to understand more about their role in promoting improved eating, drinking and communication. The children's parents can also benefit from such input. Wherever possible, in-school training should be offered to the people who feed the children and those who prepare the food.

Involve catering staff in the training to explain how what they provide and how it is presented are fundamental to the success or failure of any feeding programme. A child cannot learn to chew on liquidized food. Dieticians, therapists and school staff can all help to include the catering department in training sessions. Experience has shown that, in many cases, such intervention has had a dramatic effect on kitchen staff who are often unaware of how valuable their contribution can be. Knowing how they can help makes their job more interesting and rewarding.

POSITIONING

This has been covered in Chapter 5. However, special consideration needs to be given to the real problems faced by school staff. 'Good' chairs, prone standers and so on are not 'good' unless the child is placed in them correctly. This requires time and practice. Supervision by a physiotherapist or occupational therapist is invaluable in ensuring that the child gets what is needed from his seating or standing provision. Where a new model is on order, the physiotherapist or occupational therapist can advise on how to make best use of the 'old' chair in the interim period.

While being aware of the importance of the child's position, we must not overlook the feeder's seating comfort. If the feeders are uncomfortable they will not be able to focus their attention on the children. On a more pessimistic note, chronic back pain leads to days away from work and may even prevent people from working. Look around the school to find chairs of different heights. Use cushions and so on to adapt chairs for feeders. Their comfort is crucial! It might be appropriate to seek advice from a physiotherapist regarding lifting and handling techniques.

WHAT TO FEED

The media regularly confront us with information regarding healthy diets, yet school children are often presented with poor-quality food of inappropriate texture and temperature, and unappetizing appearance. One way of assessing school food is to decide whether or not you would eat it.

The centralization of cooking for schools has made communication more difficult, yet, in some parts of the country, schools are able to boast well presented foods. If a freezer is available on the premises it is often easier to 'bulk cook' items required by just one or two children, to freeze and use as needed. This reduces time and cost. While limited resources are a reality, some changes are possible, given the willingness to listen and learn about the children's needs.

Liquidized food

Some children do require liquidized food. However, each type of food should be liquidized separately. This is only possible if a small blender is available. One school cook told me that foods were liquidized together because her machine could not process individual-size portions. Liquidizing foods separately takes a little longer, but how else can children learn to differentiate colours and tastes and to express preferences or dislikes?

Textured food

Mixing foods together has often been thought to be helpful. However, such combinations frequently result in choking, or pieces being swallowed whole. Uniform textures are easier to manage when chewing skills are poor.

'Chewing foods'

As the children's ability improves they require the opportunity to bite off and chew pieces of food. This is not possible if everything is mashed or chopped. Providing soft-boiled rather than mashed potato is one example of the way children can be enabled to acquire new skills. Another might involve the adult in finger-feeding dry sponge and letting the child drink the custard.

Nutrition

Advice from a dietician should be available to all schools for children with special needs. Many drugs adversely affect absorption of certain vitamins and minerals; poor fluid and fibre intake lead to constipation; feeding problems frequently result in children being very underweight. These are just some of the reasons for involving dieticians in the team caring for the pupils.

TOOTH CLEANING

As described in Chapter 9, therapeutic tooth cleaning should take place after meals.

TIME

School mealtimes are busy times. A multitude of activities are involved. Physically moving the children and positioning them correctly, eating and drinking, face and handwashing, tooth brushing and toileting require a lot of time if they are to be carried out *therapeutically*: that is, in a way that helps the child make progress.

Serious consideration is needed so that those people who decide on the time allocated to meals understand what is involved. They need to watch mealtimes, even if only on video. It is impossible to achieve optimal results if meals are rushed. At least one hour is more realistic than the 20–30 minutes that are often the norm. In some areas 'feeding' is part of the curriculum and the child's needs are included in his educational programme. Time will be required in order to follow through suggested activities.

COMMUNICATION

This was dealt with in detail in Chapter 3. It is very important that those people who feed children understand their communication needs. For example, being able to say that you want a drink before you eat is very important. It is essential that anyone feeding children understand that she must respect the children's choices. It is not fair to acknowledge someone's like of carrots and dislike of peas, but then give him peas.

Children need the opportunity to exert control over their environment. Mealtimes can provide excellent opportunities, given the appropriate circumstances.

SAFETY

The problems experienced by children with special needs make mealtimes potentially hazardous. The situation described earlier, where older pupils fed younger children, is an example of an unacceptably dangerous procedure. *Training on how to deal with choking should be given to all staff involved in feeding children.*

Similarly, policies on hygiene, vaccination against hepatitis 'B' and the use of protective gloves should be determined locally. See Chapter 7 for further information on safety issues.

HOME–SCHOOL LIAISON

Nowhere does this have greater relevance than with regard to feeding. During the pre-school years, children become used to particular routines surrounding meals. They have often been fed by just one person, usually a parent, in a particular chair in a particular room. Often, they will have become accustomed to individual attention. There may have been flexibility in time allocated to meals. They will, it is hoped, have been able to exercise some choices.

Attendance at school and the mealtime routine are major changes for any child. In some cases, there are very different ideas on how to manage the child's eating and drinking. Parents may use different positioning; sadly, it is often the case that social services will only provide one chair. Children may eat different sorts of foods at home. This is particularly true for families from some ethnic minority backgrounds. In order to make this transition as smooth as possible, the following strategies might be considered.

1 At least one member of the school staff visits the child before he starts school to allow them to get to know each other and see how mealtimes have been managed.

2 One person is designated the 'key feeder' and is responsible for maintaining good liaison and seeking advice as appropriate.

3 Parents are invited into school to see how mealtimes are organized and to discuss their child's needs.

4 Therapists working in schools also see the child at home to provide carry-over.

5 Where home visiting may be particularly difficult, as for example in rural areas, one member of staff visits and makes a video of the mealtime to show to other school staff. Similarly, videos of the children eating in school can be shown to parents. This may be necessary if the presence of parents alters children's behaviour in school, and vice versa.

6 Parents going into school during a child's first weeks there, to demonstrate how he is usually fed, can help establish a successful transition.

A flexible, open approach between the parents and school staff is essential if the parents are to be successfully included in the team who care for their child.

Carry-over of 'feeding programmes'

The term 'feeding programmes' is perhaps unfortunate, as it seems to imply a regimented attitude to passively feeding children. It might be more appropriate to find an alternative, such as simply 'Improving John's mealtime'. In order for any such guidelines to work, they must be clear, concise and understood; that is, the feeder should appreciate why certain 'dos' and 'do nots' are there. The list of suggestions needs to be fairly short — pages of notes are easy to overlook. A simple one-line comment under headings such as the following is far easier to follow:

Position	
Communication	
Likes/Dislikes	
Equipment	
Dietary Information (a) Must have (b) Can't have	
Independence	

This is particularly important in situations where an unfamiliar person has to feed a child. The staff need to know what feeding equipment is available in school. Photographs are invaluable. I have found *Polaroid* cameras very helpful, as they capture something and then reproduce it in seconds. I would always photograph the main feeder doing something well — not a visiting member of staff. We learn best from our own experiences and it is encouraging to see oneself achieving success.

Resources

Lack of resources is a real problem for everyone in the fields of health and education. Adequate funding is seldom the reality. It is therefore worth contacting local fund-raising groups, as well as local stores which may 'adopt' a particular school and raise money for it. Supermarkets and food manufacturers will often provide specific foods known to be useful for the development of eating and drinking skills.

Children can benefit enormously from their eating and drinking experiences in school. It is vital that every person involved in the process works as part of a team to foster a positive, forward-thinking and therapeutic approach.

CONCLUSION

Enabling a child to thrive and grow is an essential part of his care. This book has aimed to show how feeding a child in a *therapeutic* manner can help him to develop skills in many areas, notably oral movement and communication. Eating and drinking involve many skills and effective teamwork is crucial to appropriate management. I hope that the suggestions offered in this book will provide the foundation for a happier and more successful mealtime situation for the child and the person who is feeding him.

Remember to ask yourself, **Whose meal is it**?

LIST OF
EQUIPMENT

Bottles

Haberman Feeder
Athrodax Surgical Ltd
Great Western Court
Ashburton Industrial Estate
Ross-on-Wye
Herefordshire HR9 7XP
United Kingdom
Tel: 01989 566669

Medela Inc
4610 Prime Parkway
PO Box 660
McHenry
Illinois 60051–0660
United States of America
Tel: +800 435 8316

Playtex
Branches of Boots the Chemist,
Childrens World, Mothercare and other
high street stores in the United
Kingdom. Most large drugstores in the
USA.

Rosti Bottle
Mrs Robertson
6 Blenheim Close
Danbury
Chelmsford
Essex CM3 4NE
United Kingdom

Cups

Avent Cups
Branches of Boots the Chemist,
Childrens World, Mothercare and other
high street stores in the United
Kingdom.

Also from:
Heinz Baby Club
Cherry Tree Rd
Watford
Herts WD2 5SH
United Kingdom

Cheyne Cup
S.K. Engineering
Unit 13a
Pivington Mill
Egerton Road
Pluckley
Ashford
Kent TN27 0PG
United Kingdom
Tel: 01233 840085

Doidy Cup
Smith & Nephew Homecraft Ltd
Lowmoor Road Industrial Estate
Kirkby-in-Ashfield
Notts NG17 7JZ
United Kingdom
Tel: 01623 754047

Polythene & Bickipegs Ltd
43–47 Jopps Lane
Aberdeen
Scotland AB1 1BX
United Kingdom

North Coast Medical Inc
187 Stauffer Boulevard
San Jose
California 95125–1042
United States of America

MagMag Cup
Caretime Ltd
Tradelink House
25 Beethoven Street
London W10 4LG
United Kingdom

Nottingham Rehab
17 Ludlow Hill Road
West Bridgford
Nottingham NG2 6HD
United Kingdom

Sammons Inc
PO Box 386
Western Springs
Illinois 60558–0386
United States of America
Tel: +800 323 5547

Tommee Tippee Cup
Branches of Boots the Chemist,
Childrens World, Mothercare and other
high street stores in the UK.

Variflow Beaker
Branches of Mothercare

Dental Training

NUK dental training set
Baby Orthodontic Products
PO Box 288
West Byfleet
Weybridge
Surrey KT14 6HG
United Kingdom

North Coast Medical Inc
187 Stauffer Boulevard
San Jose
California 95125–1042
United States of America

Sammons Inc
PO Box 386
Western Springs
Illinois 60558–0386
United States of America
Tel +800 323 5547

Pigeon Trainer Toothbrush Set
Caretime Ltd
Tradelink House
25 Beethoven Street
London W10 4LG
United Kingdom

Spoons

Bone Spoons
Mrs J. Barnes
The Horn Shop
3 Crag Brow
Bowness-on-Windermere
LE23 3BX
United Kingdom
Tel: 01539 444519

JA Preston Corp
Dept 1249
PO Box 89
Jackson
Mississippi 49204–0089
United States of America
Tel: +800 631 7277

Sammons Inc
PO Box 386
Western Springs
Illinois 60558–0386
United States of America
Tel: +800 323 5547

Cheyne Spoon
S.K. Engineering
Unit 13a
Pivington Mill
Egerton Road
Pluckley
Ashford
Kent TN27 0PG
United Kingdom
Tel: 01233 840085

Plastic Weaning Spoon
Boots the Chemist, Childrens World,
Mothercare and the
Heinz Baby Club
Cherry Tree Rd
Watford
Herts WD2 5SH
United Kingdom

JA Preston Corp
Dept 1249
PO Box 89
Jackson
Mississippi 49204–0089
United States of America
Tel: +800 631 7277

Sammons Inc
PO Box 386
Westem Springs
Illinois 60558–0386
United States of America
Tel: +800 323 5547

Theraspoon
Kapitex Healthcare Ltd
Freepost
LS22 4YY
United Kingdom
Tel: 01937 580796

Soft-Bite Spoon
The First Years—Boots the Chemist,
Childrens World and the
Heinz Baby Club
Cherry Tree Rd
Watford
Herts WD2 5SH
United Kingdom

North Coast Medical Inc
187 Stauffer Boulevard
San Jose
Califomia 95125–1042
United States of America

Spoons to facilitate independent/assisted feeding
Nottingham Rehab
17 Ludlow Hill Road
West Bridgford
Nottingham NG2 6HD
United Kingdom

Smith & Nephew Homecraft Ltd
Lowmoor Road Industrial Estate
Kirkby-in-Ashfield
Nottinghamshire NG17 7JZ
United Kingdom
Tel: 01623 754047

Miscellaneous
Non-slip Mats
Nottingham Rehab
17 Ludlow Hill Road
West Bridgford
Nottingham NG2 6HD
United Kingdom

Plate Guard
Nottingham Rehab
17 Ludlow Hill Road
West Bridgford
Nottingham NG2 6HD
United Kingdom

JA Preston Corp
Dept 1249
Jackson
Mississippi 49204–0089
United States of America
Tel: +800 631 7277

Sammons Inc
PO Box 386
Western Springs
Illinois 60558–0386
United States of America
Tel: +800 323 5547

Straws
Available with *MagMag* and *Avent Systems*

Pat Saunders Drinking Straw
Winslow Press Ltd
Telford Road
Bicester
Oxon OX6 0TS
United Kingdom
Tel: 01869 244644

Sammons Inc
PO Box 386
Western Springs
Illinois 60558–0386
United States of America
Tel: +800 323 5547

Travel Band
Boots the Chemist in the UK

US Range
New Visions
Route 1
Box 175–S
Faber VA 22938
United States of America
Tel: +804 361 2285

Aids to independent eating
Handy One-Robotic Aid
Rehab Robotics Ltd
Suite 3.3
Keele University
Science Park
Keele
Staffordshire ST5 5BG
United Kingdom

Neater-eater
Michaelis Engineering Ltd
13 Spencer Road
Buxton
Derbyshire SK17 9DT
United Kingdom

Clothes for children with physical disability
Special Clothes for Special Children
PO Box 4220
Alexandria
Virginia 22303
United States of America

EXAMPLES OF DIFFERENT TEXTURED FOOD & DRINK

Please note that these are guidelines. Caution should be exercised when selecting food or drink for children.

'Bite and stay firm'

Sweet

Dried bananas — whole not brittle 'chips'
Dried peaches
Dried pears
Dried apricots
Dehydrated fruit straps (health food shops)
Liquorice sticks
Bikkipegs

Savoury

Dried meat, eg. biltong
Dried fish (oriental stores)

'Bite and dissolve'

Sweet

Sponge finger (boudoir) biscuits
Wafer biscuits
Dry *Puffed Wheat* cereal
Sugar Puffs
Cheerios (cereal)
Ice cream wafers
Rice paper
Meringues
Sponge cakes

Savoury

Wotsits
Cracottes
Prawn crackers
Quavers
Skips

'Bite and chew easily'

Sweet

Ripe peeled pears (fresh or tinned)
Ripe peeled nectarines
Ripe peeled fresh peaches
Cooked peeled apples
Cooked peeled pears

Savoury

Ripe peeled avocados
Soft cooked potatoes
Soft cooked carrots
Soft cooked parsnips
Soft cooked swedes
Pieces of paté
Crumbly cheeses, eg. caerphilly
Wholemeal bread (not granary)
Soft (filleted) fish
Soft (skinned) poultry
Soft pieces of pasta (no sauce)

Thick liquid (should be completely smooth)

Milk-based

Smooth drinking yogurt
Custard
Semolina
Milk liquidized with fresh fruit
Cheese sauce
Melted ice cream
Fromage frais
Quark

Water-based

Fruit/vegetable purée
Liquidized soups
Tomato juice
Carrot juice

Other

Provamel soya-based dessert, various flavours (health food shops)

NB *It is particularly important to take great care when offering firm foods. Refer to pages 59–60, which describe how to make a food pouch.*

PRODUCT
INFORMATION

Dairy free (United Kingdom)

'Cheese/cheese spread' *Fromsoya, Green Dragon, Marigold*

Confectionery *Plamil non-dairy carob bar*

'Ice cream' *Berrydales, Dayvilles, Elysia, Genice, Granose, Ice Dream, Marinelli, So-Good*

Margarines and spreads *DP Pure, Golden Rose, Granose, Outline, Sainsbury's Dairy Free, Suma, Tomor, Vitaquell*

Soya desserts *Granose, Provamel, Sojal, Unisoy*

Soya milks *Bonsoy, Granose, Plamil, Provamel, So-Good, Sojal, Sunrise, Unisoy*

Soya yogurt *Granose, So-Good*

Tofu *Cauldron, Granose Organic, Paul's, Mori-nu*

Dairy free (United States of America)

'Cheese/cheese spread' *Soymage (no caseinates; truly nondairy), Tofu Rella, Soya Kaas*

Confectionery *Tropical Source candy bars, Health Valley granola bars, fruit bars, rice bran and oat bran bars, Glenny's fruit drops, Sunlight/Sunspire carob raisins and carob peanuts*

'Ice cream' *Rice Dream (Imagine Foods), Tofutti, Ice Bean, Living Lightly*

Margarines and spreads *Farm Soy Dairy, Spectrum Naturals, Natural Food Store Soy Bean Margarine, Nonna Lena's flavoured dips and spreads*

Soya desserts *Dream Pudding (Imagine Foods), Amazake Pudding (Grainaissance)*

Soya milks *Edensoy (Eden Foods), Westsoy (Westbrae Natural Foods), Vitasoy, Rice Dream, Pacific Foods Organic Soy Beverage*

Soya yogurt *Farm Soy Dairy, White Wave Dairyless*

Tofu *Farm Soy Dairy, Tree of Life, White Wave Soyfoods, The Soy Deli, NaSoya*

Recipes and product information regarding special diets

American Dietetic Association
216W Jackson Blvd
Suite 800
Chicago
Illinois 60606
United States of America

Consumer Nutrition Hotline:
1-800-366-1655

Berrydales
5 Lawn Road
London NW3 2XS
United Kingdom
Tel: 0171-722 2866

Nutrition Education Association
PO Box 20301
3647 Glen Haven
Houston
Texas 77225
United States of America
Tel: 1-713-665-21946

Supermarket nutrition services

Asda
Customer Services Dept
Asda Stores Ltd
Asda House
Great Wilson Street
Leeds LS11 5AD
United Kingdom
Tel: 01132 435435

Somerfield
Customer Relations
Somerfield House
Whitchurch Lane
Bristol BS14 0TJ
United Kingdom

Marks & Spencer
Marks & Spencer Plc
47 Baker Street
London WlA lDN
United Kingdom
Tel: 0171-935 4422

Publix Super Markets
Customer Relations
PO Box 407
Lakeland
Florida 33802
United States of America
Tel: 1-813-688-1188

Safeway
Safeway Stores Plc
Nutrition Advice Service
6 Millington Road
Hayes
Middx UB3 4AY
United Kingdom

Sainsbury
Customer Services
J Sainsbury plc
Stamford House
Stamford Street
London SEl 9LL
United Kingdom
Tel: 0171-921 6000

Tesco
Tesco House
PO Box 18
Delamare Road
Cheshunt
Herts EN8 9SL
United Kingdom

Waitrose
Nutritional Advice Service
Southern Industrial Area
Bracknell
Berks RG12 8YA
United Kingdom
Tel: 01344 424680

USEFUL
ADDRESSES

United Kingdom

Association of Paediatric Physiotherapists
Mrs M Lee
15 Ropemaker Road
Rotherhithe
London SE16 1QG

The Association for Rehabilitation of Communication and Oral Skills
209B Worcester Road
Malvern
Worcestershire
WR14 1SP
Tel: 01684 576795

Bobath Centre
Bradbury House
250 East End Road
London N2 8AU
Tel: 0181-444 3355

Bobath Cymru
19 Park Road
Whitchurch
Cardiff CF4 7BP
Wales
Tel: 01222 522600

British Association of Occupational Therapists
6–8 Marshalsea Road
London SE1 1HL
Tel: 0171-357 6480

British Dietetic Association
7th Floor
Elizabeth House
22 Suffolk Street Queensway
Birmingham B1 1LS
Tel: 0121-643 5483

British Institute for Sensory Integration
12 Carnarvon Road
Barnet
Herts
EN5 4LU

The Centre for Cerebral Palsy
63 Cheyne Walk
London SW3 5LT

The Chartered Society of Physiotherapy
14 Bedford Row
London WC1R 4ED
Tel: 0171-242 1941

Royal College of Speech and Language Therapists
7 Bath Place
Rivington Street
London EC2A 3DR
Tel: 0171-613 3855

Disabled Living Foundation
380-384 Harrow Road
London W9 2HU
Tel: 0171-289 6111

Dysautonomia Society of Great Britain
22 Oakwood Avenue
Borehamwood
Herts WD6 1SR

First Aid Courses
Contact the local (United Kingdom)
branches of:
St John Ambulance Association
St Andrews Ambulance Association
The British Red Cross
Colleges of Further Education

Irish Sensory Integration Association
Rosemary Shields
Occupational Therapy Department
Cooper Street Clinic
91 Cooper Street
Belfast BT13 2LJ
Northern Ireland

National Association of Paediatric Occupational Therapists
Newcommen Centre
Guys Hospital
St Thomas Street
London SE1 9RT

The National Deaf-Blind Rubella Association (Sense)
11–13 Clifton Terrace
Finsbury Park
London N4 3SR

Royal National Institute for the Blind
224 Great Portland Street
London W1N 6AA
Tel: 0171-388 1266

Royal National Institute for Deaf People
19-23 Featherstone Street
London EC17 8SL
Tel: 0171 296 8000

Sense Family Advisory Service
Sense West
Princess Royal Centre
4 Church Road
Edgbaston
Birmingham B15 3TD
Tel: 0121-456 1564

Sense Family Centre
(South East Region)
86 Cleveland Road
Ealing
London W13 OHE
Tel: 0181-991 0513

Sense Scotland
168 Dunbarton Road
Dunbarton
Partick
Glasgow G11 6XE
Tel: 0141 334 9675

Sensory Integration Association UK
3 Brickfield Cottages
Somerleyton
Suffolk NR32 5QW

Spastics Society for People with Cerebral Palsy
12 Park Crescent
London W1N 4EQ
Tel:0171-636 5020
Fax: 0171-436 0931

Study Group on Perception (UK)
Occupational Therapy Department
Frimley Childrens Centre
Church Road
Frimley
Camberley
Surrey TU16 5AD

United States of America

American Association of the Deaf-Blind
814 Thayer Avenue
Room 300
Silver Spring
Maryland 20910

American Council of the Blind
1155 15th Street NW
Suite 720
Washington DC 20005

American Deafness and Rehabilitation Association
PO Box 251554
Little Rock
Arkansas 72225

American Disability Association
2121 8th Avenue N
Suite 1623
Birmingham
Alabama 35203

American Foundation for the Blind
151,West 16th Street
New York 10011

American Occupational Therapy Association
1383 Piccard Drive
PO Box 1725
Rockville
Maryland 20849–1725

American Physical Therapy Association
1111 North Fairfax Street
Alexandria
Virginia 22314

American Speech-Language-Hearing Association
10801 Rockville Pike
Rockville
Maryland 20852

Clearinghouse on Disability Information
US Department of Education
Office of Special Education and
Rehabilitative Services
Switzer Building
Room 3132
Washington DC 20202–2524

Dysautonomia Foundation
20 East 46th Street
3rd Floor
New York 10017

First Aid Courses
Contact the local (USA) branches of:
American Red Cross National
Headquarters
431 18th Street NW
Washington DC 20006

Multidisciplinary Institute for Neuropsychological Development
48 Garden Street
Cambridge
Massachusetts 02138

National Association for Independent Living
Independent Association
55 City Hall Plaza
Brockton
Massachusetts 02401

National Association for the Visually Handicapped, Inc
3201 Balboa Street
San Francisco
Califomia 94121

National Association of the Deaf
814 Thayer Avenue
Silver Spring
Maryland 20910

National Therapeutic Recreation Society
2775 South Quincy Street
Suite 300
Arlington
Virginia 22206

Smith & Nephew Rolyan Inc
One Quality Drive
PO Box 105
Germantown
Wisconsin 53022

US Physical Therapy Association
1803 Avon Lane
Arlington Heights
Illinois 60004

United Cerebral Palsy Associations
1552 K Street NW
Suite 1112
Washington DC 20005

READING LIST
& VIDEO
PRESENTATIONS

Anderson C, *Feeding—A Guide to Assessment and Intervention with Handicapped Children*, Jordanhill College of Education, Glasgow, 1983.

Anderson J & G, *Topsy & Tim meet the Dentist*, Blackie & Son Ltd, London, 1988.

Arvedson JC & Brodsky I (ed), *Paediatric Swallowing and Feeding - Assessment & Management*, Whurr Publishers Ltd, London, 1993.

Ayres Dr A J, *Sensory Integration and the Child*, Western Psychological Services USA, California, 1983.

Blind Children's Centre, *Let's Eat,* 4120 Marathon Street, Los Angeles, California, 90092.

Bobath B & K, *Motor Development in the Different Types of Cerebral Palsy*, Heinemann, London, 1982.

Boehme R, *Approach to Treatment of the Baby*, Therapy Skill Builders, Arizona, 1990.

Boehme R, *Developing Mid-Range Control and Function in Children with Fluctuating Muscle Tone*, Therapy Skill Builders, Arizona, 1990.

Boehme R, *The Hypotonic Child*, Therapy Skill Builders, Arizona, 1990.

Carroll L, *Mealtimes for Children with Cerebral Palsy*, The Centre for Cerebral Palsy, London, l991.

Chailey Heritage Team, *Eating and Drinking Skills for the Child with Cerebral Palsy*, North Chailey, Nr Lewes, 1992.

Evans-Morris Dr S, *Pre-speech Assessment Scale*, JA Preston Corporation, New Jersey, 1982.

Evans-Morris Dr S & Dunn Klein M, *Pre-Feeding Skills*, Therapy Skill Builders, Arizona, 1987.

Finnie N, *Handling the Young Cerebral Palsied Child at Home*, Heinemann, London, 1974.

Green Dr C, *Toddler Taming*, Century Hutchinson Ltd, London, 1986.

Groher M E (ed), *Dysphagia 2E*, Butterworth-Heinemann, London, 1992.

Hill S, *Family*, Penguin, London, year unknown.

Johnson H & Scott A, *The Practical Approach to Saliva Control*, Communication Skill Builders, USA, 1993.

Levitt S, *Treatment of Cerebral Palsy and Motor Delay*, Blackwell Scientific Publications, London, 1977.

Logemann J, *Evaluation and Treatment of Swallowing Disorders*, Pro-ed, Austin, Texas, 1983.

Morse E, *My Child Won't Eat*, Penguin Paperback, Harmondsworth, 1988.

Rosenthal S (ed), *Dysphagia & the Child with Development Disabilities*, Singular Publishing Group, Inc., USA, 1994.

Tuchman DN, *Disorders of Feeding & Swallowing in Infants & Children*, Singular Publishing Group, Inc., USA, 1993.

Wolf & Glass, *Feeding & Swallowing Disorders in Infancy*, The Psychological Corporation.

Videos

St John Ambulance Association, 'Breath of Life', video demonstrating infant resuscitation. Available from St John Supplies, Priory House, St Johns Lane, London EC1M 4DA. Tel: 0171-251 0004

St John Ambulance Association, *First Aid Manual*, Dorling Kindersley, London, 1993.

Bobath Centre, 'Bobath Approach to the Treatment of Children with Cerebral Palsy', Parts 1 and 2—video presentations.

GLOSSARY

OF TERMS

Abduction   Movement of the limbs away from the mid-line of the body.

Adduction   Movement of the limbs towards the mid-line of the body.

Alignment   The relative position of the head and body; that is, the head is lined up with the body, not at an angle to it.

Aspirate   To inhale, as in aspirating food, which usually results in choking as the food 'goes down the wrong way'.

Asymmetrical   One side of the body different from the other.

Ataxic   No balance, jerky.

Athetosis   A type of cerebral palsy in which the child has uncontrolled and involuntary movements.

Auditory defensiveness   Showing a noxious response to sound.

Barium swallow (modified)   A procedure in which a small amount of liquid barium and paste and biscuit containing barium are drunk or eaten while being filmed and viewed simultaneously.

Bite reflex   Clamping down on anything introduced into the mouth.

Body awareness   Knowledge of one's body, in terms both of the idea of its different parts and of their relation to one another.

Cerebral palsy   A non-progressive but changing disorder of posture and movement; a condition resulting from damage to or maldevelopment of the brain.

Cough reflex   The protective closure of the vocal cords within the larynx to prevent food or liquid from entering the airway. It is a normal protective mechanism present throughout life. The child with cerebral palsy may have an inefficient cough reflex; that is, it may be weak or indeed absent, which increases the risk of aspiration.

Desensitization   See normalizing sensation.

Distractible   Not able to concentrate.

Dystonic   Subject to sudden change in muscle tone, between low and very high.

Elongation   Lengthening.

Extension   Straightening of any part of the body.

Eye contact   Eye-to-eye contact.

Facilitation   A handling technique which makes it possible or easier for the child to move or to tolerate stimulation.

Flexion   Bending of any part of the body.

Floppy   Loose, as the result of decreased muscle tone (see hypotonicity).

Gag reflex   A normal protective mechanism present throughout life, occurring in response to stimulation in the mouth. Individuals vary in sensitivity. The reflex is particularly sensitive in young babies and in children who do not chew very well. It may be

(1)   hypersensitive — ie is stimulated too easily, as when a child gags when food touches the lips;

(2)   hyposensitive — ie is not stimulated as quickly as normal, as in a hypotonic (floppy) child who is unable to react quickly enough to food or drink at the back of the mouth;

(3)   absent — ie not present: this is dangerous as food or drink may enter the airway;

(4)   delayed/suppressed — ie child needs to gag but abnormal muscle tone inhibits this; signs include the child's eyes watering, blinking or glazing over.

Gastrostomy   A method of feeding directly into the stomach via a tube, positioned on the abdomen (stomach).

Handling   Holding and moving with or without the help of the child.

Head control   Ability to control the position of the head.

Hypersensitivity   Increased sensitivity to touch (most common) but can also be to sound, smell or other sensation.

Hyposensitivity   Decreased sensitivity to touch (most common) but can also be to sound, smell or other sensation.

Hypotonicity   Decreased muscle tone preventing maintenance of posture against gravity; that is, there is difficulty in starting a movement because of lack of fixation.

Inhibition   A handling technique which is used to reduce abnormal muscle tightness and discourage or prevent abnormal patterns of movement from occurring, thus facilitating more normal movement.

Involuntary movements   Unintended movements.

Jaw control   See oral control.

Key points of control   Parts of the body from which abnormal movement and level and distribution of muscle tone in the rest of the body can be influenced.

Larynx   Voice box.

Mid-line   In the middle.

Motivation   Making child want to do something, innate drive to achieve.

Motor   Relating to body movement or posture.

Muscle tone   The state of tension in muscles at rest and when we move.

Normalizing sensation   The process through which a child is helped to tolerate stimulation without overreacting or underreacting to it.

Occupational therapy   Treatment given to help the child towards the greatest possible independence in daily living; may include advice on perception.

Oesophagus   Gullet, passage through which food passes to the stomach.

Oral   Related to the mouth.

Oral control   The use of a person's hand, arm or body to support or facilitate head and mouth stability or movement of another person.

Oral defensiveness   Showing a noxious response to stimulation in and/or around the mouth.

Oral–motor   Movement of the mouth: ie tongue, lips, soft palate.

Passive   That which is done to the child without his help or co-operation.

Patterns of movement   In every movement or change of posture the brain stimulates muscles to work in co-ordinated groups, ie in patterns.

Perception   The process of organizing and interpreting the sensations an individual receives from stimuli.

Physiotherapy   The treatment of disorders of movement.

Postural drainage   Positioning used to aid draining of secretions from the lungs.

Posture   Position from which the child starts a movement.

Prone   The body position with the face and stomach downward.

Proprioception   The sensations from the muscles and joints. Proprioceptive input tells the brain when and how the muscles are contracting or stretching and when and how the joints are bending, extending, being pulled or compressed. This information enables the brain to know where each part of the body is and how it is moving.

Quadriplegia   A type of cerebral palsy in which the whole body is affected.

Reflex   An innate and automatic response to sensory input. For example, we have reflexes to withdraw from pain, we blink to protect our eyes, cough to clear the airway, and so on. A reflex is beyond a person's control.

Reflux   The mechanism of gastro-oesophageal reflux is not clearly understood. One of the explanations is that the muscle fibres of the diaphragm, which function as a sphincter at the lower end of the oesophagus (gullet), fail to act in a co-ordinated manner, which allows backward flow of stomach contents back up to the oesophagus and pharynx. If the child with cerebral palsy has increased muscle tone in the abdominal muscles this will encourage reflux. Hip flexion will have a similar effect, therefore careful positioning after meals is very important.

Reinforce   React in such a way as to make a behaviour likely to be repeated.

Rooting reflex   Searching movement of mouth for teat or nipple following touch to the lips or cheeks.

Sensory integration   The organization and use of sensory information before birth and throughout the life span: the nervous system's process of assimilating and organizing sensory information for functional use.

Sensory–motor experience   The feeling of one's own movements.

Soft palate   Continuation of hard palate (roof of mouth); moves visibly when mouth is opened wide and person says "ah". Its upward movement prevents food or drink entering the nose during swallowing.

Spasm   Sudden tightening of muscles.

Spasticity   Resistance to movement. Child feels stiff to the adult handling him because of high muscle tone.

Speech and language therapy   Treatment given to develop communication and eating and drinking skills.

Stability   Being still in a controlled way.

Sucking pads   Fatty tissue within the cheeks which helps the infant to suck.

Suckle   'Suck–swallow' pattern seen in young infant.

Suctioning   A method of chest clearing using a thin tube via the airway.

Supine   The body position with the face and stomach upward.

Swallow   This involves both voluntary and involuntary movement. There are three stages: *Oral stage* — in which the food is chewed and formed into a cohesive bolus (lump) drenched in saliva. It is propelled backwards along the tongue and finally, by strong backward humping of the tongue, it is projected backwards into the pharynx. This phase involves voluntary movement. *Pharyngeal stage* — this begins once the swallow reflex has been activated at the end of the oral stage. This is involuntary. Breathing is halted throughout this stage and resumed at the end of it. During this stage, the soft palate elevates to close off the nasal airway. The larynx elevates, the vocal cords adduct and the epiglottis moves down over the larynx to protect the airway. The bolus is squeezed down past the relaxed cricopharyngeal sphincter and enters the oesophagus (gullet). *Oesophageal stage* — this final stage is involuntary. The bolus moves down the oesophagus through the relaxed gastro-oesophageal sphincter and enters the stomach. Digestion now begins. For a full description see **Langley J**, *Working with Swallowing Disorders*, Winslow Press Ltd, Bicester, 1988 and **Logemann J**, *Evaluation and Treatment of Swallowing Disorders*, Pro-ed, Texas, USA, 1983.

Symmetrical   Both sides equal.

Tactile defensiveness   Showing a noxious response to touch.

Tapping   Chest tapping is used to clear secretions from the lungs.

Tone   Firmness of muscles.

Tongue thrust   Pushing out of the tongue where there is an increase in muscle tone.

Trunk   The body as distinct from the limbs.

Videofluoroscopy   A radiographic investigation in which a radio-opaque substance (barium) is incorporated into small quantities of food and drink and is photographically recorded and simultaneously viewed on its passage from the mouth to the stomach.

INDEX

Figures in *italics* refer to illustrations

gastrostomy 79–80
gesture 15
glossary 110–112
gloves 50, 54, 82, 100
gums
    cleaning 82
    (*also see* dental care)

handling
    importance of 27
head control 39
health visitor 34
hearing impairment 30, 39, 46, 96
hepatitis B 50, 100
hygiene
    in food preparation 75
    in stimulating the mouth 54,
        82
hypersensitivity 52
hyposensitivity 52
hypotonic child 25, 31, 40, 52

icing
    use of 90
independence 45, 69–70, 95

jaw (*also see* oral)
    rotatory movement 8
    stability 56
    vertical (up) movement 6, 8,
        40

key-worker 36

laxative 77
lighting
    appropriateness of 46
lips
    closure 6, 8, 10, 54, 87
    upper lip movement 8
liquid
    recommended daily intake 76

thickened, examples of 76
thickened, use of 76

mess
    opportunity to make 69
    problem of making 69
mouth
    closure 56, 58, 59, 65
    to communicate 15
mouthing 7
movement
    normal development of 25
munching 7
muscle tone
    decreased 25
    definition of 25
    fluctuating 26
    increased 25, 27, 40
muslin pouch 62, 62

nasogastric tube 79–80
neck
    cushion 32, 49, 58
    elongation of 32
noise
    effect of 30, 46, 96
nurse 34
nutrition 47, 49, 71–80, 99

obesity 77
occupational therapist 34–35
oral (*also see* mouth)
    control 56–57
    defensiveness 52
ophthalmologist 35
orthopaedic surgeon 35
orthotist 36

parents
    importance of 34
    needs of 34, 35
    problems experienced by 1–5

perception 52
physiotherapist 34
plastic surgeon 36
play
    pretend 10, 11, 56, 62
    with food 10, 56
positioning
    for eating/drinking 29–33, 37,
        49, 65–66, 92, 98
postural drainage 50
practical exercises 7, 8, 26, 29,
        38, 39, 40, 45, 46, 51, 54, 86,
        92
preparation
    of food 49, 70, 94
prone stander 29, 30
psychiatrist 35
psychologist 35

quantity
    (food/drink) effect of 71–76

radiographer 36
radiologist 36, 50
rate of feeding 38
reflux 31, 37
religious considerations 9, 48
retching (*see* gag reflex)
rooting reflex 6

safety (*see* choking)
    issues 37
    precautions 50
saliva
    control (*see* dribbling)
    function of 86
    production of 86
schools
    particular issues relevant to
        96–101
self-feeding
    (*see* independence)

semi-solids
    introduction of 6
sensation
    normalizing 53–56
sensory defensiveness 52–53
sensory input 52, 89
sensory integration 53
sensory overload 52
sitting
    for eating/drinking 31–33
smell 41, 93
social aspects of eating/drinking
        12, 20, 48, 95
social worker 35
spasm 60, 61, 96
spastic child 25, 40
speech 10, 11, 15, 27
speech and language therapist 34
speed of feeding 38
spitting 84, 84
spoons
    assessment of 45
    feeding with 64–65
    selection of 45
    use of 45
standing
    for eating/drinking 30–31, 33
stimuli
    auditory 41
    tactile 41
    visual 41
straw
    use of 8, 68–69
sucking
    development of 6
    improving 61
    normal 6
    pads 40
suckle 6
suctioning 36, 50
swallowing 6
swimming 87